# Healing Massage Techniques

## Holistic, Classic, and Emerging Methods

# Healing Massage Techniques

## Holistic, Classic, and Emerging Methods

**Frances Tappan, Ed.D., M.A.**
Associate Dean (retired)
School of Allied Health Professionals
University of Connecticut
Storrs, Connecticut

*Foreword to the First Edition by*
**Joseph Yao**

*Prologue by*
**Michael Zito, M.S., R.P.T.**

**APPLETON & LANGE**
Norwalk, Connecticut/San Mateo, California

0-8385-3655-7

89  90  91  92  /  10  9  8  7  6  5  4  3  2

Prentice-Hall International (UK) Limited, *London*
Prentice-Hall of Australia Pty. Limited, *Sydney*
Prentice-Hall Canada, Inc., *Toronto*
Prentice-Hall Hispanoamericana, S.A., *Mexico*
Prentice-Hall of India Private Limited, *New Delhi*
Prentice-Hall of Japan, Inc., *Tokyo*
Simon & Schuster Asia Pte. Ltd., *Singapore*
Editora Prentice-Hall do Brasil Ltda., *Rio de Janeiro*
Prentice-Hall, *Englewood Cliffs, New Jersey*

**Library of Congress Cataloging-in-Publication Data**

Tappan, Frances M.
    Healing massage techniques : holistic, classic, and emerging
methods / by Frances Tappan ; with a foreword by Joseph Yao. — 2nd
ed.
        p.    cm.
    Bibliography: p.
    Includes index.
    ISBN 0-8385-3655-7
    1. Massage.  2. Acupressure.  I. Title.
    [DNLM:  1. Massage—methods.  WB 537 T174h]
RM721.T2178   1988
615.8′22—dc19
DNLM/DLC
for Library of Congress                                     88-14559
                                                              CIP

Production Editor: Mary Beth Miller
Designer: M. Chandler Martylewski, Steven M. Byrum
Cover Design: Robert Kopelman
Front and Back Cover Kirlian Photographs by Anadel Schnip of Norwichton, Connecticut

PRINTED IN THE UNITED STATES OF AMERICA

# Contents

# Contributors

**Beverly Kitts, B.S., R.P.T.**
Academic Director
Connecticut Center for Massage Therapy
Newington, Connecticut

**Stephen Kitts, R.M.T.**
Administrative Director
Connecticut Center of Massage Therapy
Newington, Connecticut

**Pauline E. Sasaki**
Clinical Director
Shiatsu Therapist Program
Connecticut Center for Massage Therapy
Newington, Connecticut

**Frances M. Tappan, Ed.D., M.A.**
Associate Dean (retired)
School of Allied Health Professions
University of Connecticut
Storrs, Connecticut

**Iona Marsaa Teeguarden, M.T., M.A., M.F.C.C.**
Author of *The Joy of Feeling: Bodymind® Acupressure* and *Acupressure Way of Health: Jin Shin Do®*.
Director
Jin Shin Do Foundation® for Bodymind® Acupressure
P.O. Box 1800
Idyllwild, California 92349

**Jasmine Ellen Wolf, B.A.**
Authorized Instructor and Practioner of Jin Shin Do Foundation
Certified Massage Therapist with the American Massage Therapist Association
Teacher of Jin Shin Do throughout New England based in Coventry, Connecticut

# Foreword to the First Edition

It has been my pleasure to meet and work with Dr Tappan since 1975. During that time I have developed a great respect for her knowledge and skill. There is a need today for more emphasis on the true value of massage, particularly as it involves touching the patient, an art almost forgotten in the hustle of today's treatment techniques. A few minutes of massage can be of untold value in establishing a warm relationship with the patient. It can also acquaint the person giving the treatment with the exact nature of the disorders, which can be felt by trained and sensitive fingers.

Although Eastern and Western medical philosophies differ in many ways, the similarities in their approaches to patient care are emphasized in this text, particularly as the effects of massage are related to blood flow, endocrine exchange, and the central nervous system.

Both Eastern and Western medicine are actively researching endorphins and enkephalins for relief of pain. Dr Tappan's text includes a careful research of contemporary physiological explanations for relief of pain by the use of massage, including the use of finger pressure to acupuncture points and the correlation between the overlapping areas of Bindegewebsmassage and acupuncture points.

This book is certainly inclusive of practically every known method of massage. I consider it a great contribution to all fields of medicine that use massage as a part of patient care with a human touch.

**Joseph Yao**

# Acknowledgments

It would be humanly impossible to give adequate acknowledgment to all of the many fine people who have contributed to the writing of this book. Primary recognition should be given to Lucille Daniels, whose vision and wisdom assisted the author in building a solid foundation in the form of a Master's thesis on massage.

Josephine A. Dolan, Professor Emeritus, School of Nursing, University of Connecticut, gave valuable advice concerning the use of massage in the field of nursing.

The members of the staff of the School of Physical Therapy at the University of Connecticut who willingly gave their time, energy, and personal resources deserve credit for their valuable assistance, especially Vera Kasaka, who used this material for 2 years and who made worthwhile suggestions that made this text clearer to those using it for the first time.

Words cannot express my appreciation to the people who typed, drew original sketches, and provided excellent editorial service, often working far into the night to meet the many deadlines involved in the production of this book, namely Gerri Pellecchia, Virginia Darrow, Nancy Wahnowsky, Patricia McClellan Miller, Michael Reilly, Debbie Zlotnick, and Mary Pat Fisher.

My thanks also to Dorothy McLaughlin, who was my patient and loyal companion as we studied acupuncture in Taipei, Taiwan; to Dr Min der Huang, our primary professor; to Dr Edith Pao, who made it possible for us to study in Taiwan; and to Dr Joseph Yao, Donald Courtial, and Dorothy McLaughlin for their assistance with descriptions and locations of the twenty acupuncture points used most commonly and thereby selected for study in this publication.

Steve and Beverly Kitts, as well as many of their faculty and graduates have been almost constant consultants as the new edition was being written, and for their work they deserve my thanks.

More recently the development of massage therapy as a profession has once again emphasized the personal need of people to be touched. It would be difficult for one to extend appreciation to the many people in this profession who have helped me in many, many subtle ways.

# Prologue to the Second Edition

Frances Tappan has written a timely book, rich in content, and it is an important contribution to the study of massage therapy. The author describes the methods of massage which she has become vastly familiar with for more than 30 years during her extensive experiences in the United States, Europe, and the Orient. At a time when widespread applications of soft tissue manipulations have emerged, this book provides a historical, empirical, and theoretical grounding of these techniques to the mechanical, physiologic, and neurophysiologic effects which are currently the foundation of all soft tissue manipulations.

The first of the book's five parts provides general information including a succinct overview of the history of massage; some introductory technical information, such as terminology and general massage principles; and an updated review of the effects of massage. The book's review of these effects as well as a discussion of recent research findings provide insights into the rationale for the applications of the massage techniques described later. Moreover, these effects become the common denominator which link many of today's massage approaches and facilitate an intuitive understanding of their usage.

Part II of the book systematically explains specific massage procedures and their applications. In an introductory chapter the professional role of the massage practitioner is described. Included are the basic knowledge and skill requirements which distinguish the professional from the technician, and those factors which serve to guide decisions to appropriately select and apply massage therapeutically.

Separate chapters on effleurage, pettrisage, friction, tapotement, and vibration are included. Each chapter gives the purpose of the stroke and discusses its application. Illustrations throughout this portion of the book, such as the photographs which demonstrate the specific patterns of each stroke, are used effectively. Chapters on regional applications of massage strokes and how health professionals, such as nurses, physical therapists, and others, might use these strokes are included and augment the reader's understanding of the many applications of the ubiquitous therapeutic touch.

In Part III variations of massage techniques are described both completely and perceptively. Included are Eastern and Western techniques, massage variations by select experts, emotional response approaches, and the currently popular massage techniques. Many of these chapters have been written by content authorities and add considerable dimension to the book.

Part IV consists of chapters on Eastern approaches (finger pressure techniques), including Shiatsu, Jin Shin Do, and Reflexology. Each chapter is meaningful and provides an understanding of the Eastern orientation, language, and application of massage therapy. In another chapter, Dr Tappan, who traveled to the orient in 1975 to study acupuncture, demonstrates how 20 acupuncture points can be incorporated into finger pressure massages used for healing purposes.

The Western massage systems of Albert J. Hoffa, Mary McMillan, James Cyriax, and James B. Mennell, and such popular approaches as manual lymphatic drainage, Polarity Therapy and the Trager approach are discussed in Part IV also. Before the deaths of Dr Mennell and Mary McMillan, Dr Tappan was able to consult with them to assure the accuracy of the descriptions of their methods. Elisabeth Dicke's Bindegewebmassage is discussed in more detail than previously available. The author studied these techniques at the Elisabeth Dicke School in Uberlingen, Germany, where she verified them before Dicke's death. A most informative and well-designed chapter on manual lymphatic drainage provides introductory technique descriptions but is primarily intended to create an awareness of this approach which has become increasingly popular as its applications and effects become better known.

Part V consists of a series of supplemental teaching material and case studies. It should prove to be handy for self-testing and as a reference source.

The emotional reactions to touch are also well documented by Dr Tappan. The observations, investigations, and impressions of a diverse research population assists in providing explanations for phenomena which often have been ballyhooed as mysticism. Drs Alyce and Elmer Green, at the Menninger Clinic in Topeka, Kansas, for example, have done extensive research relating to the psychosomatic approach to medicine, emphasizing stress as the principal factor producing dysfunction and pathological change in the patient. Dolores Krieger's work in demonstrating hemoglobin increases with touch is also discussed. A new chapter on "body–mind connections" effectively integrates the findings of related research with anecdotal experiences and suggests further consideration of the emotional reactions to touch.

Although myofascial release approaches have become increasingly popular today they are not directly discussed in this book. However, similar techniques with comparably described connective tissue effects are included. The Polarity technique, for example, shares procedures which are done in a similar manner to myofascial release techniques and which are used to correct restricted transverse fascial diaphragms. Both systems have roots in osteopathy and describe "energy" changes as well as observed autonomic responses. Familiarity with Polarity's concepts and techniques could augment both the study and application of myofascial release applications. In the Eastern approach of Jin Shin Do are techniques which at least resemble the osteopathic Somato emotional release, strain, and counterstrain (Lawrence Jones) techniques: A background inclusive of these earlier massage techniques could not only promote the development of skills but could provide an alternative theoretical basis for investigating heretofore unanswered questions related to the efficacy of the therapeutic touch.

Fran Tappan understands massage. Her book could be thought of as the ground substance which connects the varied massage approaches of Eastern and Western cultures and establishes a needed foundation for learning and interpreting the applications of today as well as in the future.

**Michael Zito, M.S., R.P.T.**
Associate Professor
Department of Allied Health
University of Connecticut
Storrs, Connecticut

# PART I
# General Information

# 1

# Introduction

Massage is the systematic and scientific manipulation of the soft tissues of the body. Although massage can be applied by electrical equipment such as vibrators, rollers, or hydrotherapeutic turbines, the purpose of this text is to describe those techniques that can be applied by use of the hands. Regardless of the individual touch developed by the massage therapist, these manipulations will be gliding, percussing, compressing, or vibrating in nature.

## TERMINOLOGY

An ancient Chinese book, *The Cong-Fou of the Tao-Tse*, of which a French translation appeared about a century ago, was probably the foundation of both our modern massage and of the manual Swedish movements, so admirably elaborated and systematized by Per Henrik Ling. Since the French brought Chinese massage to the West, most of the world continues to use the French terminology for massage strokes. Therefore, strokes that glide are called *effleurage*; those that knead are called *petrissage*; those that strike are called *tapotement;* those that compress are called *friction;* and those that shake or vibrate are called *vibration.*

## PURPOSES OF MASSAGE

There are innumerable situations that cause a metabolic imbalance within the soft tissues. Most of these can be treated with massage. The purpose of massage is to bring about any of the physiologic, mechanical, or psychologic effects attributed to this type of treatment. Relaxation, relief from pain, reduction of certain types of edema, and increased range of motion can be accomplished through the use of massage. Massage is usually combined with other therapeutic measures, and often provides a form of passive exercise when stretching techniques are used.

Massage will not only physiologically relieve pain and metabolically prepare the injured or involved muscles for exercise to their fullest capacity, but it will also encourage the confidence of the patient. Moreover, the massage itself enables the operator to evaluate the patient's soft tissue much more effectively than could any verbal or written report.

In addition to the treatment of injured or ill people, massage can be used to prepare healthy muscles for strenuous sports activity, or to assist the body in recovering from the aftereffects of such activity.

The Orientals teach massage to their children and feel very strongly that the exchange of such services is the responsibility of one human being to another. Dr Katsusuke Serizawa, professor at the Tokyo University of Education, has written a book on massage promoting holistic treatment.[1] He is convinced that a return to caring treatment can help save humankind from the isolation and inhumanity of the modern condition.

In addition to the wide use of massage, acupuncture is practiced in all Oriental nations. Knowledge of acupuncture is useful in the practice of massage because finger compression on the acupuncture points can be very effective. Due to the extensive publicity it has received one might think that acupuncture is the *only* Oriental method of treatment for injury or illness. Nothing could be further from the truth. Mao Tse-tung and the Communist Party of China attached great importance to the development of Chinese medicine. In 1958, during the "Great Leap Forward," the combining of Chinese and Western medicine resulted in acupuncture anesthesia, marking a great advancement in the science of acupuncture. Acupuncture is only part of traditional Oriental medicine, which is founded on a philosophy of life dealing with the interaction between the physician and the patient, the emotions of the person who is afflicted, and the stresses he or she experiences from external pressures.

It is the responsibility of those who realize how effectively massage can facilitate rehabilitation to see that patients receive this treatment. If it is not included in the physician's written prescription, often a tactful question will bring the value of massage to his or her attention.

Massage is a useful and integral part of the healing process. It should be used for psychologic, physiologic, mechanical, and reflex effects. Long before Christ, massage was used to relieve pain. A closer look at its history will help to clarify the development of massage.

---

[1]Katsusuke Serizawa. (1974). *Massage, the Oriental method* (8th ed.). San Francisco: Japan Publications.

# 2

# History of Massage

Massage probably began as soon as cave dwellers rubbed their bruises. Although the origin of Chinese medicine is lost in antiquity, therapeutic massage is assumed to have developed from folk medicine. It has many aspects in common with other Oriental traditions such as Indian herbal medicine and Persian medicine. It is believed that the art of massage was first mentioned in writing about 2000 B.C.

In 8000 B.C., the Yoga cult in India used respiratory exercises for religious and healing purposes as recorded in the Veda books of wisdom. Egyptian and Persian, as well as Japanese, medical literatures are full of references to bath treatments of various kinds and to massage. Hippocrates learned massage as well as gymnastics. Asclepiades, another eminent Greek physician, held the practice of this art in such esteem that he abandoned the use of all other medicines, relying exclusively upon massage, which he claimed effected a cure by restoring to the nutritive fluids their natural, free movement. He also made the discovery that sleep might be induced by gentle stroking.

Plutarch tells us that a century before the Christian era, Julius Caesar had himself pinched all over for neuralgia daily. It is well known that Caesar was subject to a severe nervous disorder (epilepsy), and it is more than probable that his prodigious labors were only rendered possible by the aid derived from massage. Pliny, the great Roman naturalist, had himself rubbed for the relief of chronic asthma. Arrian recommended massage for horses and dogs, asserting that it would strengthen the limbs, render the hair soft and glossy, and cleanse the skin. After giving directions for massage of the legs, abdomen, and back, he directed that the treatment should be terminated in the following peculiar manner, indicating that he understood the value of nerve stretching, at least for dogs, "Lift her up by the tail, and give her a good stretching; let her go, and she will shake herself and show that she liked the treatment."

The ancient Greeks Herodicus and Hippocrates left behind them prescriptions for massage and exercises. In 430 B.C. Hippocrates wrote, "It is necessary to rub the shoulder following reduction of a dislocated shoulder. It is necessary to rub the shoulder gently and smoothly."[1] The Greeks prescribed massage for their patients as well as for their athletes. They established elaborate bathhouses where exercises, massage, and baths were available, but these were patronized by the luxury loving to the exclusion of the health seekers. There is, in the Pergamon Museum in Berlin, a 2000-year-old alabaster relief from the palace of the Assyrian potentate, San Herib, depicting a massage treatment as realistically as one seen in clinics today.

The pathfinders of ancient medicine were almost forgotten during the Middle Ages. Not until the sixteenth century was interest renewed when Ambroise Paré sought an anatomical and physiologic foundation for mechanotherapy. From then on much was written about it, but nothing was actually done for mechanotherapy until the beginning of the last century, when medical gymnastics and massage took on a new life through the work of Per Henrik Ling of Sweden (1776–1839).

Ling was a fencing master and instructor of gymnastics. He began a study of massage after he had cured himself of rheumatism in the arm by percussions, and developed a method consisting of massage and medical gymnastics without distinguishing between the two. It often combined both in a simultaneous application on the theory that massage is a form of passive gymnastics. He based his system on physiology, which was just then emerging as a science.

Through his ardent study and dedication, Ling won acceptance for his new ideas. His method became known as "The Ling System," or "The Swedish Movement Treatment." In 1813, the first college to include massage in the curriculum, the Royal Gymnastic Central Institute, was established in Stockholm at the expense, and under the supervision, of the Swedish government. Ling's students subsequently published his theories, and, through them and the many foreign students at the Central Institute of Stockholm, Ling's system soon became known in a great part of the world; thus, today we refer to most "standard" massage as *Swedish massage*.

Between 1854 and 1918, the practice of massage developed from an obscure, unskilled trade to a field of medical health care, and the profession of *physical therapy* began. Reputable institutes of massage and medical gymnastics sprang up in Germany, Austria, and France. People suffering from rheumatism made yearly trips to the spas of Germany and France to

---

[1]Walter M. Solomon. (1950, August). What is happening to massage. *Archives of Physical Medicine*, 521–523.

take the "cure." This cure consisted of drinking gallons of mineral water, taking mineral baths, graduated exercise, and above all, massage. There was no place in America where one could get the same scientific attention. (This treatment is comparable to our present methods of salicylates, eliminating baths, graduated exercise, and massage.) It was a long time before the medical profession in England and America were willing to consider massage seriously.

About 1880, Just Marie Marcellin Lucas-Championnière claimed that in fractures, the soft tissue union as well as bony union should be considered from the start. Sir William Bennett of England was impressed with Lucas-Championnière's idea and started a revolutionary treatment with the use of massage at St. George's Hospital around 1899.

In 1900, Albert J. Hoffa published his book, *Technik der Massage*, in Germany. This book is still the most basic of all texts on massage, giving the clearest description of how to execute the stroke and advocating the procedures that underlie all modern techniques.[2]

The book by Max Bohm, *Massage, Its Principles and Techniques*,[3] which was translated by Elizabeth Gould in 1913, also includes some interpretations of Hoffa's techniques.

In 1902, Douglas Graham, a strong advocate of massage, published *A Treatise on Massage, Its History, Mode of Application and Effects*.[4] This text finally aroused the interest of the medical profession in the United States.

Sir Robert Jones, a leading orthopedic surgeon in England and president of the British Orthopedic Association, was an enthusiast for Lucas-Championnière's treatment of fractures. It was with his clinic at Southern Hospital in Liverpool that Mary McMillan was associated from 1911 to 1915. In the preface of his book, James B. Mennell writes, "To Sir Robert Jones I am indebted for the valuable opportunity of working for him at the Special Military Surgical Hospital, Shepherd's Bush: and he has now added to his many kindnesses that of writing the Introduction which follows."[5] Thus, the influence of Lucas-Championnière and Sir Robert Jones was exerted on both McMillan and Mennell.

In 1917, E. G. Bracket and Joel Goldthwait were interested in the reconstruction work that was being done among the allied nations. They were the inaugurators of the Reconstruction Department of the United States Army in the early part of 1918. Short intensive courses were arranged in order to train women to meet the demand for massage. McMillan served as chief

---

[2]For the purposes of this study, Hoffa's book was translated for the author by Miss Ruth Friedlander. Albert Hoffa. (1978). *Technik der massage* (13th ed.). Stuttgart, W. Germany: Ferdinand Enke.

[3]Max Bohm. (1913). *Massage, its principles and techniques*. Philadelphia: Lippincott.

[4]Douglas Graham. (1902). *A treatise on massage, its history, mode of application and effects*. Philadelphia: Lippincott.

[5]James B. Mennell. (1945). *Physical treatment by movement, manipulation and massage* (5th ed.). Philadelphia: Blakiston's Son.

aide at Walter Reed Army Hospital where her influence on present techniques was of fundamental importance.

McMillan received her special training in London at the National Hospital for Nervous Diseases, at St. George's Hospital with Sir William Bennett, and at St. Bartholomew's Hospital. After several years at the Southern Hospital, where she was in charge of massage and therapeutic exercises at Greenbank Cripples' Home, she came to the United States as director of Massage and Medical Gymnastics at Children's Hospital, Portland, Me. She then took over the responsibility of chief aide at Walter Reed Hospital, and instructor of special war emergency courses of Reed College Clinic for training reconstruction aides in physiotherapy at Portland, Ore. From 1921 to 1925, when her text was written, she was director of physiotherapy (courses for graduates) at Harvard Medical School.[6]

Mennell wrote his text, *Physical Treatment by Movement, Manipulation and Massage*, in 1917 during World War I. It has been revised several times; the fifth edition appeared in 1945. In the first chapter of this text, he says,

> I have had opportunities of watching various workers—English, French, Swedish, Italian, Danish—and have tried to select all that I saw good, and to discard what seemed to me to be bad, in their methods.[7]

Mennell says in his introduction that he did not intend his book to be seen as a text, but rather as what he considered the rationale of massage treatment, and an endeavor to show the importance of care and gentleness.

Mennell was a medical officer and lecturer of massage at the Training School of St. Thomas's Hospital, London, England, from 1912 to 1935. Until his death in March, 1957, he worked constantly to interest the medical field in the importance and usefulness of massage.

In 1929, Elisabeth Dicke developed an approach to massage that emphasizes the use of specific reflex zones, a system known as *Bindegewebsmassage*. Her work will be discussed in detail in Chapter 24.

Beginning in 1937, Gertrude Beard contributed to the study of massage through her teaching at Northwestern University in Evanston, Ill. From the many graduates of this school who had the benefit of her teachings, her influence on massage techniques in America today has been profound. Although none of her writings is directly quoted in this text, many of her concepts have been included.

In 1944, Harold D. Storms published an article describing a massage stroke he used for both diagnostic and therapeutic measures, particularly for fibrositic nodules. This technique (described in Chapter 11) is still widely used, particularly in Canada and Puerto Rico.

James Cyriax defines a specific, limited approach to massage, recom-

---

[6]Letter from Mary McMillan to Frances Tappan, June 19, 1948.
[7]Mennell (1945), p. 2.

mending a type of friction that goes across the fibers of the structure being treated (*see* Chapter 26). Because of his excellent illustrations and descriptions, many people in America today use this approach to massage.

In the summer issue of *The Massage Journal*, 1986, Patricia J. Benjamin notes that "Massage Therapy is an emerging profession in the 1980s."[8]

The increasing demand of people for "therapeutic massage" is a large part of a trend toward health care with a holistic approach. This trend includes a self-care philosophy of keeping the body well through exercise, nutrition, relaxation, and reduction of stress. It is now common knowledge that stress is one of the primary causes of illness, and because one of the primary results of massage *is* relaxation, people are seeking it to assist them in reducing stress. One should refer to Benjamin's very complete article concerning the history of massage if interested in more detail.

Since 1980, massage therapy has rapidly developed into a new profession. It has established a national organization, the American Massage Therapy Association, and is presently working on legislation that will help improve the image of massage as a therapeutic occupation.

The lingering false impression that connects therapeutic massage to what usually takes place in "massage parlors" has been difficult to eliminate. Massage therapy, however, has become an integral part of health care, as it well should be.

---

[8]Patricia J. Benjamin. (1986). The seeds of a profession. *The Massage Journal*, 41–47.

# 3

# General Principles of Massage

These general principles are derived from the author's experience as well as from researching the literature about other massage techniques.

Two basic principles should be kept in mind at all times. First, the operator should have knowledge of the patient's complete diagnosis, so that massage functions not as an isolated method, but as part of the patient's total treatment plan. Second, physical contact establishes a close relationship between operator and patient. This contact should be understanding and sympathetic, but never personal.

## PERSONAL APPEARANCE

The personal appearance of the operator should be above reproach. Clothing should be neat, clean, and comfortable, allowing freedom of motion.

## SURROUNDINGS

Massage can be given at almost any time or place. In the clinical office setting it is important that the room's temperature should be warm enough so that the patient, who is lying or sitting, still is comfortable.

A calm, peaceful, and cheerful atmosphere should be maintained. A tropical fish tank in the waiting room will provide a quiet yet interesting effect. In fact, if a guppy looks pregnant, people are often reluctant to leave the area! Easy-listening music will contribute to patient relaxation. Popular music, as well as some of the favorite classical pieces, has been credited with stimulating the immune system in the healing process. Making your own tapes is superior to a favorite radio station because commercials can then be eliminated, and tapes can be "tailored" to the individual needs of the patient. Massage can also be enhanced when the rhythm of the music matches the rhythm of the strokes.

In this day and age, particular emphasis should be placed on *clean air*. Not only should the NO SMOKING sign be visible and the rule enforced, but depending on the area in which the department is situated, whether it is located in or near polluted air, air-conditioning should be in use.

Neatness and cleanliness should be most evident; clean towels and sheets as well as other well-maintained equipment should be neatly arranged.

There is a developing practice for "massage breaks" provided by various companies for employees in stress-related activities. In these companies, or in stressful situations, massage can be conducted quite effectively with the subject seated in a chair, even fully clothed.

## CARE OF THE HANDS, WRISTS, AND FINGERS

The hands are all important in giving a massage. They should be washed before every treatment, and rings should not be worn because they might scratch the patient. The fingernails should be cut so short that one cannot see them if the hands are held up with the palm toward the face.

The hands should always be warm and dry before they touch the patient. If necessary, they can be warmed beneath an infrared lamp for a few moments or dried by applying powder to them. They can also be warmed by hot water or by rubbing them briskly together before touching the patient. In the early phase of learning massage, tension often causes nervous perspiration of the hands. A solution of alum and alcohol will reduce the amount of moisture and lessen the need for powder.

Many therapists develop arthritis of the fingers or wrists. Carpel tunnel syndrome can also develop if the therapist does not protect the wrist and fingers, especially when doing trigger point pressure points with deep friction or deep pressure to the acupuncture points. Any instrument similar to the handle of a broom can be used for deep pressure. Nevertheless, although this would protect the fingers, there is no substitute for the human touch.

If pain develops in the finger joints or in the wrists, immediate rest from extensive activity is necessary; and, of course, an integral part of the therapist's self-care routine should be exercises to keep the fingers strong and in normal balance.

Should injury occur from other sources, such as an accident while playing some sport, the therapist should not resume a heavy schedule of massage until the injury is well healed. Those who specialize in Bindegewebsmassage, which primarily uses the middle finger to apply pressure, often develop arthritis in that finger.

## POSTURE

Attention to good posture is essential if the operator is to avoid fatigue and backache. The weight should rest evenly on both feet with the body in good postural alignment. When massaging a large area, the weight should shift from one foot to the other. A good operator can apply pressure by a shift of body weight instead of using muscle strength.

## TREATMENT TABLE

The treatment table should be the right height to allow for correct postural balance of weight. In addition, a set of platforms ranging from 2 to 6 in. in height can be very useful. These platforms should be of adequate width and length to allow for the complete stance of the operator, who can place his or her hands on the part to be treated without leaning over or reaching up.

The treatment table should be of wood or metal with a firm pad or a mattress without springs. Even in the patient's home, one ideally should seek a firm surface such as a tabletop, and not treat the patient in a bed, which offers no firm support. There are, of course, numerous exceptions to this rule. A nurse, for example, often gives a back massage to a bedridden patient. Many equipment establishments offer excellent portable tables that are very useful for home treatment. Permanent tables are also available for clinical use.

## POSITIONING THE PATIENT

Specific positioning will be discussed with each unit; however, there are certain general precautions that should be considered. *Solid support must be given, extending distally and proximally as far as the joints on either side of the injury.*

It cannot be too greatly emphasized that the position should always be one that is comfortable for the patient. There are certain stretching positions that make use of the effect of gravity to put a slight stretch on individual muscles that might need it, but even these should not be so uncomfortable that the patient cannot relax.

In general, the part to be massaged should be elevated in order to allow gravity to assist the mechanical effects of the treatment and render the increased venous return that much easier. Exceptions to this rule will be mentioned later.

At no time should the patient have to exert muscular effort to hold the part being treated in position or to hold the draping about her- or himself. Sometimes sandbags or rolled towels may be used to brace a limb.

## DRAPING

Tight clothing should be removed and a sheet or towel used to cover the parts of the body not being treated. In arranging the draping, the patient should not be unnecessarily exposed to the point where it may cause embarrassment. He or she should be at ease to enjoy the treatment and feel confidence in the person who is about to administer this treatment.

Movements should be businesslike and the operator should assure the patient that he or she is capable and has a professional interest in the problems of the patient. The operator, of course, should never lean on the patient while reaching across the table to arrange the draping.

If the patient is unable to relax because of positioning, lack of adequate support to the part, apprehension concerning the treatment, tight or uncomfortable draping, or discomfort due to being too warm or too cold, the desirable effects of the massage may not be accomplished. Specific positions and basic supportive measures will be discussed later when the massage of each area of the body is described.

## LUBRICANTS

The purpose of a lubricant is to avoid uncomfortable friction between the hand of the operator and the skin of the patient. Older texts may suggest shaving the part to be massaged if superfluous hair interferes with the treatment, but this procedure is no longer recommended.

There are many types of lubricants. Any lanolin-based cold cream may be used because of its nonirritating qualities. Mineral oil or baby oil also may be used, according to preference. Any extra cream or oil can be cleansed from the patient with alcohol. If the primary effect of the massage has been to obtain relaxation, soap and warm water can be used instead of alcohol to remove the lubricant. Care should be taken not to stain the patient's clothes by leaving lubricants on the skin.

With dry skin, it is often best *not* to remove the lubricant. In such instances the patient can be advised to wear clothing that can be stained without concern.

When massaging stump ends, 70% alcohol is often used. In these cases, stimulation and toughening of the stump are desired.

Some patients may be allergic to a lubricant. This can usually be eliminated by changing the type of lubricant. A persistent rash should, of course, be called to the attention of a doctor.

Cocoa butter is often used on scar tissue caused by burns or where skin nutrition is indicated, but it has a higher melting point and is, therefore, more inconvenient to use. Olive oil may also be used for skin nutrition, but it becomes rancid quickly and is difficult to keep for general use.

Powder is very useful because it is not so difficult to cleanse following the treatment. An odorless powder should be used.

Some people prefer to massage with no lubricant, but if this method is used, care must be taken to be sure that the superficial hair of the skin is not pulled and that the hands of the person administering the massage are not moist.

Strong commercial ointments for "rubbing" often produce blisters if used in conjunction with heat and are more irritating to skin that has been made sensitive by serious illness or injury. Therefore, the use of such ointments is not encouraged. If such stronger ointments have been used by the patient before coming for treatment, care must be taken to wash them off prior to administering any heat or massage.

Too much lubricant prevents firm contact and the hands will only slip over the surface of the skin. It is better to have too little than too much lubricant; it remains a common error to use lubricants too generously. Many authorities advocate massage without any lubricant at all; however, this author advocates its proper usage and recommends some practice without the use of lubricant. Most professional therapists do not use scents of any kind with lubricants; occasionally, however, the use of scents may serve some psychologic purpose.

## AROMA THERAPY

*Aroma therapy* is a fairly new term for an age-old technique. The addition of various scents to massage powders or ointments can selectively influence whether the massage is relaxing, stimulating, or healing in its effect. Most people prefer no scent, which might linger on after the end of the treatment. Others may actually believe that a scent such as camphor extends their pain-relief time. They will offer such remarks as, "When I rub that stuff on at night I can go right to sleep and sleep all night!"

## FEEDBACK

The therapist will become better acquainted with the patient if attention is paid to the patient's subtle feedback. This is often not spoken, for people are shy to criticize those whom they consider specialists in a field. The therapist can therefore realize how treatment is being accepted by taking careful notice of behavior activities of the patient, who may tighten muscles rather than relax.

Ask if the pressure is too strong. The patient may turn pale and clammy—often a sign of weakness indicating that even the treatment itself is too tiring or that the patient is overly concerned with his or her condition and whether or not the massage is going to obtain expected goals.

Breathing patterns may alter. Slow, relaxed breathing by the patient may indicate acceptance. Rapid, shallow breathing may indicate concern, and treatment should be adjusted to accommodate the situation. Patients may begin to cry as they relax from severe tension, and the therapist's responsibility is to determine the cause. In the case of one patient, the therapist had located a tight nodule in the rhomboid area of the shoulder, and as treatment then centered to clear this spasm, the patient turned very pale and began to perspire. The therapist immediately inquired as to the nature of the problem. The patient was very upset and reported that the therapist had located a "lump" in his back; the patient thought all lumps were cancer. A quick and positive explanation of a fibrositic nodule relieved the patient's anxiety.

## PRESSURE AND RHYTHM

Pressure should be adjusted to the contours of the body and care should be used over bony areas. All strokes should be rhythmical. The pressure strokes should end with a swing off in a small half circle so that the rhythm will not be broken by an abrupt stop.

Consider the patient's threshold of pain or discomfort. All massage should begin lightly, even in patients who have slight injuries or who have no injuries but are being treated in an athletic situation. As the depth of the stroke increases, the operator should watch the patient carefully to be sure that the pressure is not greater than can be tolerated by the patient.

If a muscle tightens under the touch, it has probably been treated too severely or touched so lightly that it "tickles."

It is important to maintain physical contact with the patient once the treatment begins. The hands should not break contact with the skin in deep stroking and kneading except when changing areas. Even though some strokes require an actual loss of contact, the rhythm of the loss should suggest that the treatment is a continuing process. Mennell mentions in his description of superficial stroking that the stroke through the air should take the same length of time as the stroke on the body.[1]

Treatment should not be interrupted. To stop suddenly to adjust the draping, to dry the hands because they have too much lubricant on them, or to turn and talk to someone is upsetting to the patient and to the rhythmical procedure. The telephone should be answered by someone else, unless emergencies arise. Even then, the stop should not be sudden. Do not lift the hands in the middle of an effleurage stroke. Cover the patient to keep him or her warm during the interruption.

Stopping the treatment in order to move around the table or bed to treat the other side should not be done unless both legs or arms are being treated. Neither should one ask the patient to change position once the treatment has begun. One must learn how to approach the patient from al-

---

[1]James B. Mennell. (1945). *Physical treatment by movement, manipulation and massage* (5th ed.). Philadelphia: Blakiston's Son.

most any angle, since many involvements make it difficult or impossible for the patient to move about easily.

### Follow the Venous Flow

The pressure strokes should be in line with the venous flow, followed by a return stroke without pressure.

## DURATION

Treatment time is an individual decision. Contrary to older texts stating a routine or setting the amount of time allowed, modern operators follow the advice of Mendell and adjust the time to the needs of each patient.

## REST

Rest for the patient following treatment is always advised, especially in cases where the involved part is a weight-bearing limb that must be put to work as soon as the patient is ambulatory.

The length of time for this rest must be judged by the operator. If there is swelling in a dependent limb, the resting time should be long enough to permit reduction of swelling before ambulation is attempted.

## INDICATIONS

The one major indication for massage is the fact that touching of any kind is important from the moment we are born (*see* Chapter 19) until the moment we die. Jack Meager points out the importance of using massage to *prevent* injury in sports and with animals (*see* Chapters 17 and 18). However, many people do not seek massage until they have developed an ache or a pain.

It is essential for those doing massage to know when it is wise to do so. Muscles that are tense due to stress will respond well to massage. Massage alone is not as successful as that given along with relaxation techniques. Many physical therapists treat some aspects of injury or illness with massage to loosen superficial scar tissue in subacute phases and to reduce edema (*see* Chapter 4) when the cause does not indicate that massage could be dangerous. For the bedridden patient, massage may prevent decubitus ulcers from developing, particularly if the patient is unable to move due to paralysis or casting.

Massage therapy can relieve pain due to immobilization following injury. Often, due to discomfort, massage is needed to parts of the body other than the actual injury, to arms and shoulders following leg injuries, or to a painful back because of limbs placed in traction.

Tension is caused in persons by activities that overuse particular muscles, such as those with computer workers who sit at desks, musicians who practice for hours at a time, or dancers and often athletes.

## CONTRAINDICATIONS

With the emergence of alternative massage forms, it has become even more difficult to list contraindications for massage. For example, whereas it would obviously be unwise to perform Swedish massage over a malignant tumor, a form such as Polarity Therapy or Therapeutic Touch could be very helpful for stress reduction and pain management.

It is important for the professional practitioner to have a thorough background in anatomy and physiology so that he or she can research individual pathologies as they present. The *principles* of contraindications can then be applied to help ascertain if harm could be done through massage. The understanding of these principles is far more important than memorizing a long list of specific pathologies.

1. Do not use Swedish massage over any pathologic condition that might be spread along the skin, through the lymph or the blood stream.

   **Examples:** Impetigo—a skin infection usually caused by staph or strep.

   Lymphangitis—inflammation of the lymphatic vessels, sometimes called blood poisoning by the lay person.

   Malignant melanoma—a cancerous mole or tumor, which metastasizes (spreads) easily through the blood stream or lymph.

2. Do not use Swedish massage near or over any area where there is bleeding. (Other massage forms may be used for pain relief and psychologic comfort, as long as the injured area is not physically disturbed and its circulation is not increased.)

   **Examples:** Ecchymosis—a bruise.

   Whiplash or other acute injury where there is tearing of tissue—may be bleeding into the tissue during the first 24 to 48 hours after the trauma.

3. Do not use Swedish massage over areas of acute inflammation. (Friction techniques may be treatment of choice in chronic stage.)

   **Examples:** Appendicitis.

   Rheumatoid arthritis—over acutely inflamed joints.

   Acute febrile conditions.

4. Research carefully, including getting physician's recommendation, when working with clients with disorders of the circulatory system.

   **Examples:** Cardiac arrhythmias or carotid bruit—avoid lateral and anterior neck.

   Phlebitis, or thrombophlebitis—elevate area, avoid completely except for application of hydrotherapy as recommended by physician.

   Severe atherosclerosis.

   Severe varicose veins.

5. Be especially careful in areas of abnormal sensation.

   **Examples:** Decreased sensation due to stroke, diabetes, medication (muscle relaxants)—client cannot give you accurate feedback on depth and may have abnormal vasomotor response to your work.

   Hyperesthesia—increased sensitivity to touch.

6. Be especially certain that you understand the anatomy and the physician's recommendations in cases where there is a loss of integrity in an area.

   **Examples:** Over recent surgery—only someone specifically trained to work with recent scar tissue should attempt this work.

   Joint replacements—be certain to check as to recommended restrictions in range of motion of replaced joints.

   Chronic sacroiliac joint subluxation—unilateral deep pressure over one ilium and not the other—may increase the subluxation.

   Severe rheumatoid arthritis (RA)—affects ligaments and joint capsule. May be very important even when RA is not acute. For example, if the odontoid ligament between C1-2 has been destroyed, the spinal cord could be injured by strong passive neck flexion.

7. Be especially careful of physician's recommendations regarding hygiene when working with a client with a compromised immune system.

   **Examples:** Receiving immunosuppressant medication following organ transplant.

   Acquired immune deficiency syndrome (AIDS).

8. Understand the pathogenesis of a symptom. For example, if a client presents with edema, it is important to know the origin. Is it related to kidney problems, venous insufficiency, arterial insufficiency or heart failure? Once the pathogenesis is understood, appropriate po-

sitioning and techniques can be selected so as to best support the health of the client and cause no harm.

Massage therapy is a valuable adjunct to regular medical care, as it reintroduces the element of touch and stress reduction, in addition to the many physical benefits already discussed. In the hands of a skilled professional, the touch may vary from light to very deep, and actually may be involved in the treatment of pathology. However, even in the hands of a young child, massage given with love and sensitivity can be very supportive and helpful to a person in need. Those who are without training and yet feel moved to serve friends or family through touch need not be afraid.

Most of the above contraindications and precautions are based on common sense. If the giver of massage is motivated by sincere concern, is gentle in giving, and is receptive and responsive to feedback from the recipient, the experience will most likely be a healthy one for both people.

## THE USE OF ICE WITH MASSAGE

A very effective way to bring blood to an area is through the application of ice. Ice applied directly to the skin, however, is too cold and too hard. Packing ice in a towel to preserve the cold temperature is fine, but as it melts, the towel leaks. A damp towel or washcloth moistened with ice water is the most comfortable, but the towel needs to be changed often. The best way to chill the area is to apply a professional ice pack that consists of a permanent package that will mold to the part as it thaws out, and is wrapped in a towel to help hold it in place.

When a part is chilled, blood races to the area. Thus, the eventual effect is an increase in circulation. This is even more effective than the application of heat.

## SUMMARY

One should avoid treating patients without complete knowledge of the diagnosis. Personal appearance should be above reproach; hands should be warm and clean; and good posture alignment is necessary. The patient should be comfortable and warm, and in a position that is functional for the operator. All tight clothing should be removed, and draping should protect the modesty of the patient. Lubricants may at times be convenient but are never absolutely necessary.

# 4

# Effects of Massage

Massage is a healing art. It is a unique way of communicating without words. By touching another person, we may communicate the fact that we *care*; we empathize and want to share our energy with that person.

Dolores Krieger, Ph.D., R.N., in 1972 proved in a controlled study that hemoglobin could be increased through the use of Therapeutic Touch.[1] Krieger writes that,

> We can help each other and we can help ourselves through Therapeutic Touch. Whether through the channeling of natural energy sources on the physical level, or the recruiting of human energy sources on the psychodynamic level, the message is clear: a new age is dawning in which we can intelligently cooperate with nature, in which we can intelligently cooperate with each other.[2]

In suggesting as an underlying drive the concept of a need to help, Krieger further states,

> A need to help wells up from the same psychodynamic depths from which arose the stimuli that guided early man not merely to mate, but to form the nuclear family in which attributes of love and caring and protection from harm were nurtured. This need to help is probably the most humane

---

[1]Dolores Krieger. (1973). The relationship of touch with intent to help or to heal, Ss in-vivo hemoglobin values: A study in personalized interactions. *Proceedings of the American Nurses Association, 9th Nursing Research Conference.* Kansas City: Author.

[2]Dolores Krieger. (1976, April). Nursing research for a new age. *Nursing Times, 72,* 1–7.

of human characteristics. It lies very close to the central motivations that bring most people into health care.[3]

Krieger's research is concerned with Therapeutic Touch, which derives, but is not the same as, the laying-on of hands. She says it is the uniquely human act of *concern* of one individual for another that is characterized by touching in an act that incorporates an intent to help or to heal the person so touched.

> To be truly therapeutic, this act must be deeply motivated in the best interests of the person who is being touched. The person doing the touching must be educable, for although the act seems quite simple, it is in fact quite complex and the toucher must be able to understand the underlying dynamics of these complexities. One must, for instance, be able to learn to recognize certain cues to subtle levels of consciousness in order to be intelligently aware of the processes, conscious and unconscious, which may be set in motion; and one must be able to develop the insight to recognize whether this mode of therapeutics is meeting the patient's needs or buttressing one's own ego structure. Therapeutic Touch is a tool frequently used by those who deliver health care, either knowledgeably or unconsciously. Since we are responsible for our acts, therefore, it behooves us to understand the basis for this particular mode of therapeutics as well as we would understand the underlying dynamics of any pharmaceuticals that might be given, or any other procedure in which we might engage ourselves.[4]

Because massage is most certainly touching, Krieger's ideas concerning the importance of the way touching is done to promote healing have a direct relationship to the touching involved in massage as one of the healing procedures.

The effects of massage are not only psychologic but also mechanical, physiologic, and reflexive in nature. By massage, stimulation is provided to the exteroceptors of the skin and proprioceptive receptors of the underlying tissues. Relief from pain is brought about through any one of these effects, or by a combination of any of them.

## ACTIVATING THE IMMUNE SYSTEM

The more one becomes familiar with Bernie Siegel's methods, the more one realizes that a loving, compassionate approach can activate the immune system toward self-healing. In 1978, Siegel attended a workshop given by Carl Simonton, an oncologist, and his wife, Barbara, a psychologist. The Simontons were teaching mental imagery for healing purposes. This impelled Sie-

---

[3]Krieger (1976), pp. 1–7.
[4]Krieger (1976), pp. 1–7.

gel toward the establishment of ECaP, a program for people with cata-strophic illnesses, be it cancer, multiple sclerosis, or acquired immune deficiency syndrome (AIDS). He studied all sorts of healing approaches and combined them into an incredibly effective healing source. The theme is that a person's emotions have a profound influence on the course of disease.

These emotions of which the patient may not be aware emerge through drawings. Skilled interpretation can help the healer understand whether the patient expects the suggested healing method to be successful.

Above all, Siegel is the kind of physician everyone would like to have. He not only teaches this method, he *is* a warm, compassionate, loving hu-man being who reflects the golden imagery of healing. If people radiate joy they will have a positive healing effect on others and help them learn to live as fully as possible for each moment of their lives.[5]

## MECHANICAL EFFECTS OF MASSAGE

Mechanically, massage assists the venous flow of blood, encourages lym-phatic flow, reduces certain types of edema, provides gentle stretching of tissue, and relieves subcutaneous scar tissue.

### Assists Venous Flow

Normally, the constant contraction of muscles as people move about pushes against the veins, pressing the blood on toward the heart. When this normal activity is inhibited by injury or illness, the resulting decreased circulation adds another complication to the already disturbed metabolism of the tis-sues involved.

The mechanical effect of deep stroking on the superficial veins in the direction of the venous flow is easily observed in many persons. The result-ing decreased venous pressure provides a favorable situation for increased arterial circulation. When capillary pressure is reduced, the potential for filtration into the extracellular spaces is decreased; thus, the load on the lymphatics is also decreased and the possibility of fibrosis is diminished.

When possible, gravity should be considered to assist, rather than in-hibit, the flow of blood within the veins. The valves within the veins prevent any backflow of blood once it has been encouraged forward. This direct mechanical effect includes mainly the more superficial veins.

### Assists Lymphatic Flow

Lymph is a viscid fluid that moves slowly through the lymphatic system. The lymphatics are, for the most part, noncontractile. Movement of lymph depends upon outside forces such as the contraction of muscles and pres-sure generated by filtration of fluid from the capillaries. Immobility due to

---

[5]Bernie S. Siegel. (1986). *Love, medicine & miracles.* New York: Harper & Row.

pain or paralysis seriously interferes with lymph drainage. The lymphatics have a lower pressure and slower flow than the venous flow.

Massage can encourage lymphatic flow, preventing the edema that often occurs with inactivity. Because lymph is viscid and moves slowly, massage strokes should be slow and rhythmical when used for this purpose. Massage is an excellent mechanical substitute when normal muscular functioning has been interrupted, but active exercise should be encouraged as soon as possible. According to Ladd, Kottke, and Blanchard, massage will increase lymphatic flow, but active exercise will do this more efficiently.[6]

### Stretches

Another mechanical effect of massage is the stretching of superficial tissues. When combined with a passive-exercise type of stretching, it will encourage the patient to relax and allow further passive stretching of a muscle that has become shortened.

### Loosens Scar Tissue

Subcutaneous scar tissue can at times be loosened by careful and persistent friction. Once it has formed, deeper scarring in connective tissue *cannot* be relieved by massage. Massage can prevent scarring *to some degree* by not allowing stagnation of tissue edema following injury, thus preventing fibrosis.

### Obesity

The old idea that obesity can be reduced by massage has been dispelled. Massage too traumatic for humans to tolerate might bruise the adipose tissue, necessitating replacement with new tissue. However, this new tissue would only be *more* adipose tissue. As a "come on" in reducing salons, massage is combined with steam baths which reduce the water content of the body through excessive perspiration, thus showing an immediate loss of weight on the salon scale. Massage can only induce a psychologic feeling of well-being for such customers.

### Muscle Mass, Strength, and Motion

Massage is ineffective in delaying loss of mass and strength following nerve injuries. It will not hasten the recovery of sensation. It will, however, accelerate voluntary and reflex action once the nerve injury has begun to recover and reenervation is present. In such cases massage should be combined with passive and active reeducational exercise.

Therefore, massage is a part of the patient's total rehabilitation program, not an independent treatment to be used by itself. Any evaluation of the usefulness of massage must consider its role in total patient care.

---

[6]M. P. Ladd, F. J. Kottke, & R. S. Blanchard. (1952, October). Studies of the effect of massage on the flow of lymph from the foreleg of the dog. *Archives of Physical Medicine, 33*, 604.

## PHYSIOLOGIC EFFECTS

The student of massage should have some understanding of the physiology of the heart and circulation, particularly the peripheral circulation and the return flow of blood and lymph, as taught in basic physiology courses.

The purpose of this discussion is to summarize and review basic physiology relating to massage.

### Metabolism

Metabolically, the muscles maintain a chemical balance through normal activity. As they contract they rid themselves of toxic products by "milking" these acids into the lymphatic and venous flow. As they contract, they assist this lymphatic and venous flow toward the heart through mechanical pressure that pushes blood and lymph through channels where valves prevent a backflow. Thus, these by-products are carried away.

As the muscles relax, fresh blood flows into them, bringing necessary nutrition to the area.

*Overactivity* disturbs this balance by not allowing sufficient relaxation time for the inflow of nutritive products. At the same time, due to exertion, toxic products are formed faster than they can be eliminated. Thus the muscle is loaded with irritant acids.

*Underactivity* also disturbs this balance by not providing the "milking" effect to assist the venous and lymphatic return. Hence, the irritant products that form within the muscles are not carried away as they should be and the muscle becomes more or less "stagnant."

Following extreme activity, these irritant acids can be hastened back into the venous return by massage. Often the "lameness" that follows abnormal activity could be lessened or prevented by massage immediately following the activity, since the muscles themselves are inhibited by fatigue.

In many situations, when partial or total muscular inactivity occurs, massage can mechanically assist the "milking" process. However, it can never replace normal muscular activity.

### Venostasis

Muscular inactivity can bring about a venostasis, particularly in the dependent limbs where gravity inhibits the normal venous return. Other causes for venostasis may be varicosity, thrombosis, or pressure on the vessels by edema within the surrounding tissues (due to local inflammation or due to the venostasis itself).

It is obvious that massage should *not* be given if there is a possibility of spreading inflammation, if there is a possibility of dislodging a thrombus, thus causing embolism, or if there is such obstruction that the mechanical assistance of massage could not improve the venous flow. Massage given *first* to the proximal aspects of an injured limb will ensure that these circulatory pathways are open enough to carry the venous flow along toward the heart.

# Edema

Edema refers to excess interstitial fluid in the tissues. Edema is not a disease, but rather the manifestation of altered physiologic function.

***Causes.*** Alterations in physiologic function that lead to edema are (1) increases in capillary filtration pressure; (2) decreases in capillary colloid osmotic pressure; (3) increases in capillary permeability; and (4) obstruction to lymph flow. Edema can occur in healthy as well as sick individuals; for example, the swelling of hands and feet that occurs in hot weather.

***Increased Capillary Pressure.*** Edema develops when an increase in capillary pressure causes excess movement of fluid from the capillary bed into the interstitial spaces. Among the factors that cause an increase in capillary pressures are (1) decreased resistance to flow through the arterioles and capillary sphincters that supply the capillary bed; (2) increased resistance to outflow at the venous end of the capillary bed; (3) increased extracellular fluid volume associated with an increase in intravascular volume; and (4) increased gravitational forces. In hives and other allergic or inflammatory conditions, localized edema develops because of a histamine-induced dilation of the precapillary sphincters and arterioles that supply the swollen area. Impaired venous outflow from the capillary causes a retrograde increase in capillary pressure. Thrombophlebitis, or the presence of venous blood clots, leads to edema of the affected part. In right-sided heart failure, blood dams up through the entire systemic venous system, causing organ congestion and edema of the dependent extremities. Increased reabsorption of sodium and water by the kidney leads to an increase in extracellular volume with an increase in capillary pressure and subsequent movement of fluid into the tissue spaces. In hot weather, dilation of the superficial blood vessels occurs and sodium and water retention increases, which causes swelling of the hands and feet. Edema of the ankles and feet becomes more pronounced during prolonged periods of standing when the forces of gravity are superimposed on the heat-induced vasodilatation and the increase in extracellular fluid volume.

***Decreased Colloid Osmotic Pressure.*** The plasma proteins exert the osmotic force that is needed to move fluid back into the capillary from the tissue spaces. Edema develops when plasma protein levels become inadequate because of abnormal losses or reduced production. The glomerulus of the kidney nephron is a network of capillaries. In certain conditions, these capillaries may become permeable to the plasma proteins. When this happens, large amounts of plasma proteins are filtered out of the blood and then lost in the urine. An excess loss of plasma proteins also occurs when large areas of skin are injured or destroyed. Edema is a common problem during the early stages of a burn, resulting from both capillary injury and loss of plasma proteins.

Plasma proteins are synthesized from amino acids. In starvation and malnutrition, edema develops because of the absence of amino acids for use in plasma protein production. In starvation, edema may actually mask the loss of tissue mass. Finally, because plasma proteins are synthesized in the liver, severe liver dysfunction causes decreased plasma protein synthesis with the development of edema and ascites. Liver disease also contributes to edema formation by causing obstruction to venous flow through the portal circulation and through impaired metabolism of hormones, such as aldosterone, which increase sodium retention.

It is now possible to measure the colloid osmotic pressure of the plasma (25.4 is normal). Infusion of albumin can be used to raise colloidal osmotic pressure as a means of restoring intravascular volume or reversing interstitial fluid losses.

***Increased Capillary Permeability.*** In situations of increased capillary permeability, the capillary pores become enlarged or the integrity of the capillary wall is destroyed. Injury due to burns, mechanical distension, inflammation, and immune responses are known to increase capillary permeability. Once an increase in capillary permeability has been established, plasma proteins and other osmotically active particles leak out into the interstitial spaces and perpetuate the accumulation of tissue fluid.

***Obstruction of Lymphatic Flow.*** The osmotically active plasma proteins and other large particles rely on the lymphatics for movement back into the circulatory system from the interstitial spaces. Lymph edema occurs when there is obstructed lymph flow. Malignant involvement of lymph structures or removal of lymph nodes at the time of cancer surgery are common causes of lymphedema. Another cause of lymphedema is infection. Elephantiasis (filariasis) is a tropical infection in which nematodes of the superfamily Filarioidea invade the lymph nodes, causing massive swelling of a body part. This infection has been reported to cause a single leg to swell to such proportions that it weighs almost as much as the rest of the body.

***Effects.*** The effects of edema are determined largely by its location. Edema of the brain, larynx, and lung is an acute, life-threatening situation. On the other hand, swelling of the hands and feet is often insidious in onset and may or may not be associated with disease. Edema may interfere with movement; it may limit motion, or cause difficulty in opening of the eyes. Edema can also be disfiguring. In terms of psychologic effects and self-concept, edema often causes a distortion of body features, creating problems in obtaining proper-fitting clothing and shoes.

At the tissue level, edema increases the distance for diffusion of oxygen, nutrients, and wastes. Edematous tissues are usually more susceptible to injury and to development of ischemic tissue damage, including pressure sores. The skin of a severely swollen finger can act as a tourniquet, shutting off the blood flow to the finger.

In chronic edema, the tissue spaces become stretched like an old balloon so that less filtration pressure is needed to push fluids into the interstitial spaces. The stretching of the tissue spaces makes correction or permanent reversal of edema difficult.

**Pitting Edema.** Pitting edema occurs when the accumulation of interstitial fluid exceeds the absorptive capacity of the tissue gel. In pitting edema, the tissue water is mobile and can be translocated with pressure exerted by a finger. Imagine, if you will, a sponge that is supersaturated with water. To test for pitting edema, the observer applies firm finger pressure to the edematous areas. Pitting edema is present if an indentation remains after the finger has been removed.

**Nonpitting Edema.** Nonpitting edema usually represents a situation in which serum proteins that have accumulated in the tissue spaces coagulate. Often, the area is firm and discolored. Brawny edema describes a type of nonpitting edema in which the skin thickens and hardens. Nonpitting edema is seen most frequently following local infection or trauma.

**Assessment.** Methods for assessing edema comprise visual inspection, including the use of digital pressure to determine the degree of pitting that is present. Pitting edema is evaluated on a scale of plus 1 to plus 4. Daily weight is also a useful index of interstitial fluid gain. A third assessment measure involves measuring the circumference of an extremity (or the abdomen).

**Treatment.** The treatment of edema is usually directed toward (1) maintaining life in situations in which the swelling involves vital structures; (2) correcting or controlling the cause; and (3) preventing tissue injury. Diuretic therapy is often used to treat edema. The reader is again reminded that edema is not always associated with disease and that normal compensatory increases in tissue fluid may respond to such simple measures as elevating the feet.

Elastic support stockings and sleeves are applied to increase the resistance to the outward flow of fluid from the capillary. These support devices are often prescribed in situations such as lymphatic or venous obstruction and are most efficient if applied before the tissue spaces have filled with fluid, for instance, in the morning, before the effects of gravity have caused fluid to move into the ankles.

**Accumulation of Fluid in the Serous Cavities.** The serous cavities are potential spaces located in strategic body areas where there is continual movement of body structures—the joints, the pericardial sac, and the pleural cavity. The exchange of extracellular fluid between the capillaries, the interstitial spaces, and the potential space of the serous cavity is similar to capillary exchange mechanisms that exist elsewhere in the body. The potential spaces are closely linked with lymphatic drainage systems. The milking action of the moving structures continually forces fluid and plasma proteins back into the circulation, keeping these cavities empty. One of the factors that contributes to fluid accumulation in a potential space is obstruction to lymph flow.

The preface *hydro* may be used to indicate the presence of excessive fluid, as in hydrothorax, which means excessive fluid in the pleural cavity. Or the term *effusion* may be used, as in pleural effusion, referring to an accumulation of fluid in the pleural cavity.

The fluid accumulated in a serous cavity may be either serous or exudative. A common cause of fluid accumulation in serous cavities is infection. In infection, white cells and cellular debris collect and obstruct lymph flow, causing osmotically active proteins to accumulate. A second cause of fluid accumulation is a malignant tumor; malignant tumors may invade the lymph channels that drain the serous cavity, and thus contribute to fluid accumulation.

*Ascites* is an accumulation of fluid in the peritoneal cavity. Because of its location in relation to the portal circulation, the peritoneal cavity is more susceptible to excess fluid accumulation than are other body cavities. This is so because anytime pressure in the liver sinusoids increases significantly, serum exudes through the capillaries on the surface of the liver and passes into the peritoneal cavity. Congestive heart failure, cirrhosis, and carcinoma of the liver are examples of conditions that obstruct hepatic blood flow and cause fluid to move into the peritoneal cavity. Because the portal vein receives blood from the peritoneal surface, portal hypertension creates an increase in the filtration pressure of the capillaries that line the peritoneal cavity.

Excess fluid may be aspirated or removed from a serous cavity. The term *paracentesis* refers to removal of fluid through a puncture site. Usually a needle or similar instrument is inserted into the cavity and the fluid is withdrawn. Analysis of the fluid for the presence of infectious organisms and malignant cells often aids in diagnosis of the disease responsible for the fluid accumulation.

These types of edema should *not* be treated with massage, unless in a specific instance a physician gives careful instructions for an unusual situation. There are, however, certain types of edema where massage can be of some assistance. Already mentioned is the venostasis caused by muscular inactivity, which may be due to paralysis, injury, or illness. If there is no actual obstruction (such as thrombus) and the edema is caused only by the inactivity of the part, there can be no harm in massaging edema from the foot and ankle. An example is a well-healed fracture of the femur which is not yet able to bear weight, but the leg is allowed to hang down in a dependent position with little or no muscular activity. Without adequate instruction for nonweight-bearing exercises and advice for part-time elevation of the leg (so that gravity can assist the venous return), massage alone will be of little assistance. Massage is not in itself a total treatment, but contributes an important part to the total treatment.

In cases of recent injury, where edema is evident due to torn tissues and internal bleeding, massage to the injured area would only encourage further bleeding and more swelling. If massage is indicated at all, it should be given only to areas proximal to the injury, or given so superficially that no further injury would be caused. One should *never* give massage to any area exhibiting this type of edema unless ordered by a physician, who will indicate when sufficient healing has taken place to tolerate such treatment.

*Summary.*  In summary, edema occurs in healthy as well as sick individuals. The physiologic mechanisms that predispose to edema formation are (1) increased capillary pressure; (2) decreased capillary colloidal osmotic pressure; (3) increased capillary permeability; and (4) obstruction of lymphatic flow. The effect that edema exerts on body function is determined by its location—cerebral edema can be a life-threatening situation, whereas swollen feet can be a normal discomfort that accompanies hot weather.[7]

## REFLEX EFFECTS

Sir James MacKenzie defines the reflex process as, "that vital process which is concerned in the reception of a stimulus by one organ or tissue and its conduction to another organ, which on receiving a stimulus produces the effect."[8] In massage, the hands stimulate the sensory receptors of the skin and subcutaneous tissues, causing reflex effects. The stimuli pass along the afferent fibers of the peripheral nervous system to the spinal cord; from there, it is conceivable that these stimuli may disperse through the central and autonomic nervous systems, producing various effects in any zone supplied from the same segment of the spinal cord. Some of these effects are capillary vasodilation or constriction, relaxation or stimulation of voluntary muscle contraction, and gooseflesh. In addition, there is the possible sedation or stimulation of sensory reception with sedation or stimulation of pain. In extreme cases reflex effects may be severe. They could cause nausea, vomiting, and depression of the heart's action with resulting pallor and sweating.

On this principle Elisabeth Dicke organized the specific routine described in her text, *Meine Bindegewebsmassage.* If these viscerocutaneous

---

[7]From Carol Mattson Porth. (1986). *Pathophysiology: Concepts of altered health states* (2nd ed.). Philadelphia: Lippincott, p. 442, with permission.
[8]J. MacKenzie. (1923). *Angina pectoris.* London: Henry Frowde and Hodder and Stoughton, p. 47.

effects are possible it can be seen that beneficial effects from massage of specific zones could be produced with controlled results.

Miriam Jacobs discussed the reflex effects of massage as follows:

The increased circulation by way of improved superficial venous and lymphatic flow is an effect of deep pressure produced by stroking or compression movements. Mechanical pressure from stroking movements probably also produces direct effects upon the capillaries resulting in capillary contraction as seen in the "white" reaction following mechanical stimulation of the skin. It is said to be of capillary origin and is not dependent upon nerves. According to the standard physiology texts, it may be a direct response of the capillaries to irritation or to some substance liberated as a result of the mechanical stimulus. With firmer pressure, a "red" reaction appears. This is the result of capillary dilation and is not dependent upon nervous mechanisms. Stronger stimuli or repeated stimuli produce a "red flare" and is due to dilation of the arteriole. It is thought that dilation of the arteriole may be due to a local axon reflex mechanism (1). With an intense stimulus (which is not considered a desirable massage procedure in this country) a wheal may be formed. This "triple response" red reaction, red flare and wheal formation is believed to be brought about by a diffusion of a substance liberated by the cells of the skin in response to mechanical stimulation. The substance bears a resemblance to histamine in its effects; capillary dilation by its direct effects, arteriole dilation by the axon reflex, and finally a wheal due to the increased capillary permeability and the release of fluid.

The existence of vasoconstrictor nerve fibers which increase the tone of the arterioles is unquestioned. Their cells of origin are located in the intermediolateral column of gray matter of the thoracic and upper lumbar cord and their fibers pass via the anterior roots to synapse in the chain ganglia via the white rami; they rejoin the segmental spinal nerves via the gray rami to be distributed to the vessels of the skin and muscles. The anatomy of the vasodilator fibers is confusing and debatable. The vasoconstrictor fibers are limited for the most part to the sympathetic system; the vasodilator fibers may not be restricted to the parasympathetic system as is often described. Barron suggests that vasodilator fibers are distributed not only via the parasympathetic outflow but they are also found comingled with the vasoconstrictor fibers of the sympathetic outflow (2). Another group of vasodilator fibers are said to be intermingled with the afferents of the spinal nerves. At the periphery, an afferent fiber from a receptor in the skin may give off a collateral to the arterioles of the vascular bed of the skin. Thus, local stimulation of the skin sets up (in addition to the afferent impulses to the central nervous system) an axon reflex that acts upon the arterioles. That vasodilation does follow experimentally produced antidromic stimulation (causing impulses to flow back to the receptor) of the dorsal root is generally accepted. The question that is debated is whether impulses are normally set up in the central ends of the dorsal root afferents, for neural control of the blood vessels of the skin. Such an antidromic effect could explain the effects of massage; i.e., peripheral stimulation of the sensory afferents resulting in reflex dilation of the arterioles of the muscles and vascular bed of the skin.

Bayliss has shown that stimulation of the sensory afferent nerves from the limbs in animals brings about vasodilation due to inhibition of the local vasoconstrictors as well as excitation of the local vasodilators, an effect comparable to reciprocal innervation seen in skeletal muscle (2). Thus the blood supply increased by the sensory stimulation of massage may be a combination of excitation of the vasodilators and inhibition of the vasoconstrictors.

Barron suggests that evidence is also accumulating which indicates that there are pressure sensitive fibers intermingled in other nerves of the blood vessels of the skin and viscera which if activated bring about a fall in blood pressure through vasodilatation of the splanchnic region (2). He further states that stimulation of the sciatic or other mixed nerves by cooling, activation by weak stimuli or mechanical stimuli may cause vasodilation of the splanchnic area (2). This might explain some of the visceral effects claimed by the advocates of Bindegewebsmassage which may be termed a weak stimulus (3).

Deep pain following ischemia resulting from sustained muscle contraction may be relieved by massage through the improved circulation afforded by, 1) the mechanical pressure on superficial venous and lymphatic channels, and 2) reflex dilatation through stimulation of the cutaneous afferents mediating touch and pressure. Another possibility for the relief of pain may be mediated through another mechanism. The stretch or tension, placed on the tendons and fascia surrounding the muscles during the stretching and compression movements, as in petrissage, may have an inhibitory effect on sustained muscle contraction. It is a well known fact that a "cramped muscle" can be relaxed by stretching it or by deep kneading. Impulses from the tendon sensory organs (probably Golgi tendon organs) and perhaps also from the fascia and adjacent joint structures, which are activated by stretch, produce powerful central inhibition of the neurons controlling that muscle. This effect has been called the inverse myotatic reflex (4). Relaxation and the relief of pain of sustained muscle contraction by massage and traction might possibly be explained on this basis.[9]

## References for Miriam Jacobs's Article

1. Bard, Philip. (1956). *Medical physiology.* St. Louis: Mosby, p. 158.
2. Barron, D. J. (1955). Physiology of the organs of circulation of the blood and lymph. Sec. VI. In J. F. Fulton (Ed.), *Textbook of physiology.* Philadelphia: Saunders, pp. 566, 755.
3. Ebner, M. (1956, August). Peripheral circulatory disturbances: Treatment by massage of connective tissues in reflex zones. *British Physical Medicine, 19,* 176.
4. Lloyd, D. P. C. (1955). Principles of nervous activity. Sec. I. In J. F. Fulton (Ed.), *Textbook of physiology.* Philadelphia: Saunders, p. 104.

---

[9]Miram Jacobs. (1960, February). Massage for the relief of pain: Anatomical and physiological considerations. *Physical Therapy Review, 40,* 96–97. Reprinted with the kind permission of Miriam Jacobs and the *Physical Therapy Review.*

## EFFECTS OF MASSAGE ON THE SKIN

Since the hands contact the skin when massage is conducted, the effects of this treatment on the skin should be considered. One of the major effects is the contact this pressure makes with the sensory nerve endings. Usually, massage is sedative and these effects are, therefore, beneficial. If, however, there is a nerve injury present that makes these sensory nerve endings extremely hypersensitive, so sensitive in fact that massage does not bring sedation but only increases the pain of the patient, it is then contraindicated. It would not be given unless the operator could lower the pain threshold of the patient by an extremely technical approach. Occasionally these patients can tolerate a firm contact better than a superficial one, and if such were the case, continued massage might be indicated.

The condition of the skin following extreme injury is often abnormal. Parts that have been in a cast will have layers of dead skin under which tender, new skin has developed. In cases where the skin has been burned, massage would not be indicated until adequate scar tissue has formed. Decision as to when this type of tissue (and it may be a skin graft) may be treated is made by the physician in charge.

Because the skin helps remove excretory products its pores must be kept open. If there are layers of dead skin inhibiting the normal functions of skin, they can best be removed by first subjecting the part to whirlpool, followed by massage. The friction of massage will create heat which invites perspiration and increases sebaceous excretions. The skin also carries out a certain amount of respiration (exchanging carbon dioxide and oxygen) and can be assisted in this by massaging the part that has been in a cast where the normal functioning of the skin has been inhibited. Massage in these cases helps the skin return to normal function.

Occasionally a patient's skin will react to massage by breaking out or showing infections of the hair follicles. In the presence of such infections, massage is discontinued until reordered by the physician, or the type of lubricant is changed, or occasionally massage without lubricant is given.

## SUMMARY

Massage increases venous and lymphatic flow, reduces certain types of edema, provides stretching of tissue, relieves subcutaneous scar tissue, improves nutrition through the skin by the application of special lubricants, increases perspiration, thus removing excretory products, helps to remove dry scaly skin following casting, and assists soft tissue toward normal metabolic balance. In addition, there are reflex effects from the stimulation of sensory receptors of the skin and subcutaneous tissues.

# 5

# The Body–Mind Connection

The art of healing is a two-way street. A massage given by one who includes the patient as a partner will be remarkably more effective than that given as a mere technique of body manipulation. One who devotes total attention by communicating concern, empathy, and a sincere desire to promote the healing process will spur a patient to participate in the effort toward regaining health.

The mutual objective of both the therapist and the patient is to replace the patient's dependency with a collaborative effort on the part of both patient and operator. To establish this relationship, the patient must participate in discussions that include an exchange of ideas, rather than simply receive instructions given by the operator. Such an approach will strengthen positive attitudes and exclude feelings of despair.

A pleasant atmosphere, the exchange of laughter, a sense of strength or determination, and feelings of love will strongly encourage the human body toward its own constant search for homeostasis. The body itself will then produce more complicated and comprehensive chemotherapy than is available at any medical center in the world; be it via Eastern or Western medical approaches (*see* Endorphins in Chapter 6).

While giving massage, one can encourage the patient to understand the potential source of healing in his or her own consciousness. The patient can be encouraged not to be helpless, passive, depressed, or desperate, but rather capable and active in his or her own treatments. According to Bernie Siegel, "The body heals, not the therapy . . . the body can utilize any form of energy for healing . . . even plain water—as long as the patient believes in it."[1] Everyone wants to love and be loved. Skillful encouragement can stimulate the human body's defense and healing mechanisms.

---

[1]Bernie S. Siegel. (1986). *Love, medicine & miracles*. New York: Harper & Row, p. 129.

Current research done with plants, animals, and human beings is proving that positive effects are possible through the "laying-on of hands." "Lay thy hand upon it" goes as far back as Sushruta Samhita. In an experiment conducted in 1964, Bernard Grad used barley seeds that had been soaked in saline to stimulate a "sick" condition. Oskar Estebany worked with Grad as a "healer" and held flasks of water as he would were he doing laying-on of hands. An identical saline flask of barley seeds was not treated by the laying-on of hands. The seeds held by Estebany sprouted more quickly, grew taller, and contained more chlorophyll.[2]

In the book *The Secret Life of Plants*,[3] Peter Tompkins and Christopher Bird recorded how Cleve Backster proved without doubt that plants respond if touched with affection. By using lie detector equipment he confirmed Grad's studies that plants respond to loving care and soft music in a positive way. Conversely, they respond negatively to hard rock music and feelings of hate.

In fact, Backster conceived a threat that he would burn an actual leaf of a dracaenia plant to which his lie machine galvanometer was attached. The *instant* he got the picture of "flame" in his mind and before he could move for a match, there was a dramatic change in the tracing pattern on the graph in the form of a prolonged upward sweep of the recording pen. Backster had not moved either toward the plant or toward the recording machine. Could the plant have been reading his mind?

In fact, there is a lamp on the market, the base of which holds potted plants. When a leaf is touched, a light bulb will go on. A three-way light bulb will cycle through low, medium, and high to off, each time a leaf is touched. During demonstrations, the light refused to go on although the pot had been recently watered. After several people had tried to transfer enough energy to light the bulb and had failed, the demonstrator suggested that the plant must be thirsty and requested a glass of water that was handed to her in a paper cup. Before the plant had even been touched (in fact, the cup of water was at least 4 in. from the plant), the lamp light turned on. The demonstrator pulled her hand back and the light went off, again before being touched at all. This plant was considered further proof of Backster's theory that plants respond to human thought or mental intent.

In Eastern cultures the transference of attitudes between the healer and the subject is believed to occur via a state of matter for which Western culture has neither a word nor a concept. It is called *prana* in Sanskrit. The nearest translation in English is *vitality* or *vigor*. The Chinese call it *Chi*, which translates as *energy*. Regardless of what it is called, however, this phenomenon refers to the balanced functioning of the human body and the vital life force of energy, which keeps people in good physiologic and psy-

[2]Bernard Grad, et al. (1964). A telekinetic effect on plant growth, Part 2. Experiments involving treatment with saline in stoppered bottles. *International Journal of Parapsychology, 6,* 473.
[3]Peter Tompkins & Christopher Bird. (1973). *The secret life of plants.* New York: Avon, p. 19.

chologic health. Think of the world as having a "collective consciousness" and join the "self" to that strength. Lessen thoughts of yourself as "only one." Advocates of this concept believe that positive energy can be transferred from the healer to the patient through touch (via any medical approach—pulse reading, acupuncture, or more modern medical methods) to return the patient to normal health. They also believe that it is absolutely necessary for the patient to have faith in the healer and to possess a strong will to get well. Siegel tells of a woman in the hospital who visualized her x-ray therapy as a "golden beam of sunshine entering her body." He also believes that people set up defenses against sharing their innermost feelings with anyone. If they feel their ability to love shriveling up, they create a vicious cycle that leads to further despair. Anger can be a cry for help.[4]

Massage is one of the best ways to transfer the strong healing energy from the giver to the receiver.

Krieger's recent controlled study proved that therapeutic touch, or the laying-on of hands, is a uniquely effective human act. Her results showed significant measurable changes in hemoglobin values. By touching with the intent to help or heal, the patient would feel heat within the area beneath the hand. Patients reported feeling profoundly relaxed and having a sense of well-being.[5]

In *Anatomy of an Illness as perceived by the patient*,[6] Norman Cousins records how he became, with his doctor, William Hitzig, a participant in the accomplishment of his own recovery. Together they proved that a cheerful atmosphere and an open-minded exchange of ideas related to recovery actually reduced the high sedimentation rate causing his illness. He achieved an almost complete recovery and returned to functional health.

Such attitudes do not develop without concentrated effort on the part of the healer and the one desiring to be healed. All patients are individuals with problems, physical problems that create mental attitudes that may vary all the way from complete rejection of treatment to complete cooperation. Before treating a patient, explain what the treatment will accomplish. Always try to find out what the patient is thinking and feeling by listening more than talking. Work *with* the patient. Inspire the patient's confidence with a positive attitude that implies that your knowledge and skill are available. This also means that the healer cannot afford to display any personal, negative feelings regardless of anger or rudeness on the part of the patient. A healer's firm, controlled strength of character can guide the patient toward acceptance and belief that the treatment is beneficial.

Sick people become dependent on others in many cases. The therapist should strive to replace patient dependency with self-sufficiency; identify

---

[4]Bernie S. Siegel. (1986, April). Love medicine. *New Age Journal, 50*, 52.

[5]Dolores Krieger. (1976, April). Nursing research for a new age. *Nursing Times, 72*, 1.

[6]Norman Cousins. (1979). *Anatomy of an illness as perceived by the patient: Reflections on healing and regeneration.* New York: Norton, p. 48.

important life goals; and eliminate the patient's feelings of despair and loneliness. This can be done by exchanging ideas and sharing knowledge.

Fear can be depressing, if not deadly, so everything possible should be done to strengthen positive attitudes. The atmosphere should always be pleasant. Direct sunlight from windows with a pleasant view is helpful. Tropical fish tanks and tranquil music help the surroundings to be peaceful and interesting. Harmonious relationships should be encouraged.

Illness often follows a crisis that creates a sense of hopelessness and despair. It is interesting to note that each person is ultimately responsible for both the illness and the recovery. People from all aspects of health care can help each *body* in their own special way, but no *body* is going to *heal* unless the body itself *decides* to heal.

The therapist can be most effective by taking careful note of the whole patient at the first moment of contact. Body language can speak louder than words. You can determine how a person feels by the look in her eyes, the way he holds his head, the slump of her shoulders, his tone of voice, or even by noting whether he or she seems to feel happy or depressed.

Above all, the therapist needs to convince the patient that the treatment being given is going to bring relief from pain and recovery from depression. Each patient needs loving support, understanding, a purpose for living, and some sense of satisfaction related to the efforts put forth on his or her behalf.

If massage is to be "healing," both the giver and the receiver will be comfortable with the idea that shared energy and unconditional love provide strong motivation toward healing. Look for the love and light in people. This exchange of healing energy comes in many forms other than massage. It can occur through group concerns with people who share similar problems. People can interact negatively or positively. Never forget, "four hugs a day keep the blues away." People can accept or reject, even subconsciously, the positive energy being extended in their surrounding external environment.

As a therapist who is involved with touching, one is in a particularly advantageous position to transfer healing energy by the way in which art, skill, and knowledge are shown during treatment. To help the therapist know what the patient is thinking, questions such as, "Do you enjoy what you are doing?" should be asked. Each person being treated should be understood by the therapist as much as possible, relative to the importance of feeling relaxed and at peace, in order to encourage the caring, loving energy of healing.

There was the case of a dying cancer patient who said to her therapist, "I wish someone would talk to me about dying! My doctor always changes the subject and my own family refuses to talk about it."

The therapist giving massage answered, "You can say anything you want to me."

For the remainder of the treatment they discussed death and the patient's basic beliefs in positive terms. One person can be terrified under stressful situations, and die of a heart attack; another person can face the same situation with no terror at all. Those people who are often terrified or angry about situations that occur are less likely to respond to the extension of healing energy.

If you ask seriously ill patients if they would like to live, many of them will say, "No." Nevertheless, ask the same seriously ill people if they would like to live and *feel physically well and active,* and most of them will say, "Yes!" Do not make the mistake of assuming that all seriously ill people really want to die.

An understanding of death at any age is a must for all therapists, because so many dying people truly need the loving touch of massage.

Our DNA inhibits or permits physiologic responses. The human body and mind are ONE. People may enhance their *basic gene inheritance* by using their energy to cope with stress. All therapists should be aware of their own individual status, know whether they are at peace at work and in their other external environments, and whether they are balanced enough to enhance the healing energy they hope to deliver. They should know how to "center" their own energy toward the well-being of their patients.

In class or group sessions, good energy "breaks" are essential to keep the positive energy flowing. One technique is to interrupt the presentation and interject without introduction, "Reach out and touch someone." Responses in the group will vary all the way from those who refuse to touch or to be touched, to those who are not satisfied merely to touch but go beyond, even to a hug. It may take several such breaks in a large group before each member trusts the others enough to transfer any healing energy. These breaks can "sneak in" when people learn to trust, so they may be interjected as follows:

1. Reach out and touch someone.
2. Now reach out, touch someone with a warm, caring touch.
3. Find a sensitive, painful spot and touch it gently, projecting healing thoughts, and with warmth.
4. Massage the tension away from a painful area.

After asking them to "reach out and touch someone" ask each person to make a fist. Tell the person immediately nearby to open the fist. Reaction will range from those who voluntarily open their own fists to those who strongly resist having anyone try to force their fists open.

What does this tell us? People are all different, depending on their *internal* environment, and in how they respond to external stimulations.

The author has witnessed a wide range of reactions. Actually, if one is attempting to get a group of strangers into a peaceful state of mind, it is the responsibility of the leader to use instinct, observation, conversation, and careful notation of the peoples' acceptance or resistance to the idea; from that information the leader may attempt to establish a positive relationship for maximum healing results.

Those in the healing profession should realize that what they see and feel about "what's going on" is not necessarily so. All of us "perform" constantly. For example, when asked, "How do you feel today?" the typical answer is "Fine!" Actually, that person may have a splitting headache, or the flu, but is not willing to discuss it at the present time, or with that particular person.

The therapist needs to find out how a patient *really* feels *most of the time*. Loving, caring people do not always find support in their daily family or working routine. People may feel negative, or they may feel, "Just do the job! Get it done!" If so, the massage therapist will find it difficult to effect relaxation in that person.

Many a busy executive enjoys a "quick fix" massage. This could help reduce stress; it might even relax an exhausted person right into a peaceful snooze. A good therapist will realize whether a "quick fix" is enough, and advise accordingly.

Many organizations are now hiring therapists to provide "quick fixes" twice a week. The primary problem with this plan is that, soon, every employee wants a "quick fix" daily.

This procedure is too new to evaluate its permanent value toward enhanced productivity. If it contributes to employees' feeling content with and good about themselves and their work benefits, it may revolutionize the profession of massage.

All levels of the desire or need to be touched exist in a normal population. Some folks are just born to love, to be touched, hugged, held, and appreciated. If they get this in living surroundings, they are peaceful people. Others are born, or learn, to reject close contacts. They prefer to be reserved, to live "in their own closet" so to speak.

If a massage therapist who understands these differences can help such people to be less inward oriented and become more outgoing, the massage as a "stress buster" will have positive—even healing—effects. There are no "absolutes" to these ways of life. A peaceful person may desire to live, to care for loved ones, and to fulfill career goals.

Anyone could die from a heart attack when not even under stress. However, if one truly has (not pretends to have) a peaceful inner life, chances are better for a strong immune system and much greater health and healing is possible. Belief systems are powerful enough to cure or kill, often with dramatic effects.

Those people who stop and ask, "Would I choose to live with myself as I am right now?" and answer "Yes," usually have a super immune system that works to keep the body in balance, and these people are the easiest to relax with massage techniques.

One should ask of oneself, "If I had only a year to live, what would I do?" A peaceful soul would reply, "Maximize good living without compulsive goals or impossible dreams. Adjust as peacefully as possible to all of life's ups and downs."

If these are not the answers, people could try to change their basic living style toward that goal. Not everyone can do this, and some who do may find it takes more energy than expected. Then the work of the giving of unconditional love to others becomes more readily received. This is the challenge of change. It is said that nothing is sure but death and taxes. Yet, there is one more thing we can be sure of, and that is change. Change can be hard to deal with. A person may want to change his or her "inner being." That is not, however, as easy as deciding to do so. Everyone looks at his or her own environment and reacts to it depending on his or her DNA (inherited genes). From birth—or even while in fetal development—change that shapes and forms character begins to occur. There are those who feel that one cannot change life patterns. Asking the question "What is your purpose in life?" could start one on the road to positive thinking. An evaluation of one's total belief system could be the beginning of change, and striving to be at peace with yourself could improve one's immune system. Massage therapists must ask themselves all these questions before they will be able to transfer healing energy to others.

It is, therefore, not how a person perceives the immediate environment, but what this means to the *inner* environment that strengthens or weakens the immune system. Some people may react to others' actions with anger, then hide that emotion and smile outwardly. Another one may yell and scream over a similar action. In the long run, the inner selves who cannot cope are the ones who will eventually kill themselves when they continue to react negatively or to frustrate themselves and thus deplete the strength of their immune system because no other course of action seems available. In short, it is not the environment outside the self that is deadly. Rather, it is the way the *inner* self feels in relation to the *outside* environment that can be damaging.

John Newbern is credited with the adage that people can be divided into three groups: "Those who make things happen, those who watch things happen, and those who wonder what happened!"[7] It is the operator's responsibility to encourage the patient to do all in his or her power to "make things happen."

## SUMMARY

It should be firmly emphasized that the terms *healing* or *the healer* do not refer to the mystical or occult. It is a proven fact that one is much more likely to achieve the balance of health and happiness with positive attitudes than with negative feelings. The importance of touch, particularly as it relates to massage, can make the difference between healing and the lack of it. Recently more emphasis has been placed on holistic methods of healing, such as control of the autonomic nervous system using imagery, love, touching, and stressing the importance of attitude.

---

[7]Krieger (1976), pp. 1–7.

# —6

# Pain Relief Through Massage

## ENDORPHINS

The physiology of pain and how to relieve it has led to the discovery of endorphins (*end*ogenous m*orphine*), which grew out of the identification of opiate receptors in the brain and other tissues. That is, sites on the cell surface specifically combine with the opiates in order to produce their characteristic biologic effects of analgesia and euphoria.

### Pain Perception

The basic sensation of hurtfulness, or pain, occurs at the level of the thalamus. In the neospinothalamic system, interconnections between the lateral thalamus and the somatosensory cortex are necessary to add precision and discrimination to the pain sensation (Fig. 6–1). Association areas of the parietal cortex are essential to the perception, or learned meaningfulness, of the pain experience. For example, if a mosquito bites a person's finger on the left hand and only the thalamus is functional, the person will complain of pain somewhere on the hand. With the primary sensory cortex functional, the person can localize the pain to the precise area on the index finger. The association cortex, however, is necessary in order to interpret the buzzing and the sensation that preceded the pain as being related to the mosquito bite.

The paleospinothalamic system projects diffusely from the intralaminar nuclei of the thalamus to large areas of the cortex and is associated with wakefulness and attention. This may explain the tremendous arousal affects of certain pain stimuli.

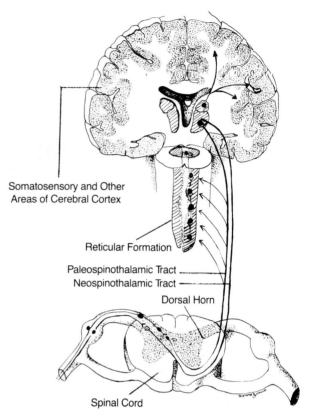

**Figure 6-1.** The spinothalamic system, one of the several ascending systems that carry pain impulses. One spinothalamic tract runs to the thalamic nuclei and has fibers that project to the somatosensory cortex. Another tract sends collateral fibers to the reticular formation and other structures, from which further fibers project to the thalamus. These fibers finally influence the hypothalamus and limbic system, as well as the cerebral cortex. *Adapted from Rodman M. J., Karch, A. M., Boyden, E. H., Smith, D. W.* Pharmacology and drug therapy in nursing (3rd ed.). *Philadelphia: Lippincott, p. 1061.*

The area in the medial thalamus (nucleus submedius), along with its projections into the limbic system, is also thought to be a possible pain center. It appears to be involved in the affective, arousal, or motivational aspects of pain.

The reticulospinal system projects bilaterally to the reticular formation of the brain stem. This system in conjunction with the collaterals of the paleospinothalamic system facilitates avoidance reflexes at all levels. It also contributes to an increase in the EEG activity associated with alertness and indirectly influences hypothalamic functions.

## Endogenous Analgesic Mechanisms

Focal stimulation of the midbrain central gray region was reported by Reynolds 4 years after the introduction of gate control theory. The analgesic level was sufficient to permit abdominal surgery, although levels of consciousness and reactions to auditory and visual stimuli remained unaffected. A few years later, opiate receptors were found to be highly concentrated in the regions of the central nervous system (CNS) where electrical stimulation produced analgesia. This led to a search for natural body substances capable of interacting with these receptors. The natural ligands, or binding molecules, for these opiate receptors are the endogenous opioid peptides (the endorphins and enkephalins), which were discovered in 1975. New therapeutic approaches to the treatment of pain were envisioned when: (1) it was discovered that these peptides exert inhibitory modulation of pain transmission; and (2) the release of endogenous opioids following CNS stimulation was correlated with patient reports of pain relief.

Endorphins (morphinelike substances) are found primarily in the amygdala, limbic system, hypothalamic–pituitary axis, and other brain stem structures. They have increased resistance to enzymatic degradation, compared with the enkephalins, and function like neurohormones. The enkephalins (in the head) are found primarily in short interneurons of the periaqueductal gray (PAG) of the midbrain, limbic system, basal ganglia, hypothalamus, and spinal cord, where they undergo rapid enzymatic degradation and may function in a manner similar to neurotransmitters.

The presence of these morphinelike substances tends to mimic the peripheral and central effects of morphine and other opiate drugs. Opiate receptors have been identified in the nervous tissue of various parts of the CNS and in the plexuses of the gastrointestinal (GI) tract. The amygdala has the greatest density of opiate receptors, followed in decreasing sequence by the hypothalamus, thalamus, and PAG of the midbrain and diencephalon.[1]

Chronic pain is as complex as the human body. The physical, psychological, and emotional must be considered in the medley of integrating the knowledge and skills of all of the medical team involved in the treatment of each case. Empathy, patience, tolerance, and faith are as necessary to treatment as improved knowledge and skills.

Massage is the one treatment that can relieve pain and can best do so when the situation is not complicated by excessive medication, such as sedatives, narcotics, analgesics, barbiturates, or alcohol. Brain neurotransmitter imbalances result from long-term use of drugs.

Massage can have its best effects by stimulating the endorphin production to reduce pain when medication for pain has become ineffective due to its overuse.

Pain is always a symptom, and the cause of the symptom is often difficult to diagnose. Many a patient has suffered real pain due to the absence of an accurate diagnosis. Often, it is precisely these people who will respond to massage therapy, primarily because "somebody cares"; some other person is giving them the caring, empathetic attention they have been denied because confused diagnosticians blame the patient, saying, "It's all in your head," or referring them for psychoanalysis.

Avram Goldstein, professor of pharmacology at Stanford University and director of the Addiction Research Foundation, Palo Alto, Calif., is a leading

---

[1]Carol Mattson Porth. (1986). *Pathophysiology: Concepts of altered health states* (2nd ed.). Philadelphia: Lippincott, p. 871.

researcher in opioid peptides (endorphins) in the pituitary and brain.[2] His investigation has been directed toward characterizing the pituitary opioid peptides that behave as typical opioid antagonists. For example, Naloxone is a synthetic drug that is a specific antagonist of endorphins and blocks their effect. Laboratory animals given Naloxone feel more intense pain than those not given the drug.

In addition, Goldstein found peptides of different molecular size could display opioid activity. He also says, "The brain is basically a chemical organ. Those many thousands of millions of brain cells talk to each other in chemical language." He calls endorphins *the morphine within*.[3]

Enkephalins are specific penopeptides belonging to the endorphin class. Enkephalins are similar to neurotransmitters. In experiments by Goldstein at the Addiction Research Center, endorphins have been shown to have an effect on mood.[4] Normal people were put in stressful, anxiety-producing situations. Some were given Naloxone, which blocks endorphins, whereas others were given a placebo. Those receiving the placebo experienced a relaxation response once the stressful situation ended; those given Naloxone remained keyed-up and anxious. This seems to demonstrate the tranquilizing effect of endorphins. Goldstein says, "Maybe we all carry our own dope around in our heads."[5]

Research into enkephalins has been a major breakthrough in bridging the gap between *acupuncture* and *neurophysiology*. The Chinese have used acupuncture for mood elevation for thousands of years, long before anyone knew about endorphins. Acupuncture (peripheral stimulation of the loci) produces analgesia. For example, accurate stimulation of the ear point, or "Lung," relieves the symptoms of drug withdrawal in animals and humans, between 10 and 30 minutes after onset of stimulation. This time lag indicates that acupuncture mechanisms involve the production and release of endogenous humeral factors.[6]

Research has been done with the transfusion of whole blood, serum, and cerebrospinal fluid in rabbits, rats, and dogs who had been given a specific acupuncture stimulation. Rabbits were given acupuncture and then bled, with their serum transfused to other rabbits. Analgesia developed in 70% of the recipients in the same limb as that of the donor. This left 30% who did not respond. Serum from nonacupunctured rabbits had no effect when transfused to other rabbits.[7]

There is still another peptide (anodynin) producing analgesia that lasts longer than enkephalins. Removal of the pituitary glands of rats results in

---

[2]Avram Goldstein. (1976, September). Opioid peptides (endorphins) in pituitary and brain. *Science, 193,* 1081.

[3]Stanford University Medical Center. (1977). The morphine within. *The Healing Arts, 7,* 7.

[4]Stanford University Medical Center (1977), p. 8.

[5]Stanford University Medical Center (1977), p. 8.

[6]P. A. M. Rogers. (1977, April). Enkephalins. *Acupuncture Research Quarterly, 1,* 64.

[7]Rogers (1977, April), p. 64.

almost complete disappearance of anodynin from blood. Researchers believe it may be involved in the activity of opiate receptors in nerves of peripheral tissues, and are studying the effects of stress, pain, sleep, and other physiologic states on the concentration of anodynin in the blood. Anodynin may be released into the bloodstream with acupuncture.

Julie Wang, in "Breaking Out of the Pain Trap,"[8] refers to other ways that acupuncture might be effective. Studies show that dietary and chemical depletion of brain serotonin levels increases sensitivity to pain. Both lack of sleep and depression are related to low serotonin. It is possible that acupuncture may have some effect on the serotonin levels within the brain.

David Mayer has performed some of the same tests on human beings at the Medical College in Virginia.

> Dr. David Mayer at the Medical College of Virginia used normal humans who were subjected to experimental pain caused by electrical stimulation of their teeth. First he showed that acupuncture did increase pain threshold. Then he administered Naloxone under double blind experimental conditions. Naloxone significantly reduced the analgesic effects of acupuncture. From this it can be concluded that acupuncture relieves pain by causing a release of enkephalins in the central nervous system.[9]

Bruce Pomeranz of the University of Toronto has shown that the electrical activity of spinal neurons is significantly diminished by acupuncture. After removing the pituitary gland from cats, Pomeranz found that acupuncture had no effect on the transmission of pain signals. Because the pituitary is a primary source of endorphin, he concluded that acupuncture needling stimulates nerves deep in the muscles to release endorphin from the pituitary, thereby producing analgesia. The effect of morphine and of endorphin can be blocked by the opiate antagonist, Naloxone.

Pomeranz believes that 30% of the patients with chronic pain who fail to respond to acupuncture do *not* have opiate receptors in the brain. This same number of people fail to respond to morphine. About 30% of all people cannot be hypnotized, probably the same people who cannot respond to acupuncture or morphine.[10]

## IMAGERY AND SUBLIMINAL TAPES

It once was thought that the autonomic nervous system, which regulates the body's organs, could not be voluntarily or consciously controlled to any significant degree. Recent evidence indicates otherwise. Psychologist Neal

---

[8]Julie Wang. (1977, July). Breaking out of the pain trap. *Psychology Today*, p. 78.
[9]Solomon Snyder. (1977, November 28). The brain's own opiates. *Chemical and Engineering News*, 35.
[10]Snyder (1977, November 28), p. 79.

E. Miller of Rockefeller University in New York has used a system of reward and punishment to demonstrate that animals can be conditioned to control autonomic processes, such as the flow of blood to various parts of the body.[11]

Human beings also can develop voluntary control of the autonomic nervous system, for example, lowering their blood pressure, by learning to control normally unconscious parts of the mind. This kind of learning usually requires visual or audible feedback, such as a flashing light or a buzzer. These cues inform the subject of his or her success, and whether or not the normally unconscious domain inside the skin is being controlled.

Although there is a line of separation between the conscious and the unconscious, the voluntary and the involuntary nervous systems, this separation apparently can shift back and forth. For example, when we learn to drive a car we focus conscious attention on every detail of muscular behavior and visual feedback. We manipulate steering wheel, gas pedal, and brakes according to what we see on the road ahead of us. Visual feedback tells us what we are doing and suggests corrections if, for example, the car heads toward a ditch. Through such feedback we learn conscious control of the striate, or voluntary, muscles. After much experience, driving becomes automatic. We then may take a long drive while thinking about something else and then wonder if we stopped at all the traffic lights.

When this behavior occurs, processes normally controlled by the conscious mind have temporarily shifted to the unconscious. When, through feedback, voluntary control is exerted over so-called involuntary processes, such as dilating and contracting the smooth muscles that control blood flow, the shift is back to the conscious domain.

Observing the early work in this field, psychologist Gardner Murphy, former head of the Menninger Foundation Research Department, Topeka, Kansas, thought that biofeedback might be useful.[12] This meant connecting monitoring equipment to visual or audible signaling devices. For example, when a thermistor was connected to a meter or a buzzer, the subject could determine whether his or her attempt to change skin temperature was succeeding by watching the meter needle or hearing the buzzer.

When biofeedback is combined with autogenic training, many people can learn to control unconscious physiologic functions more quickly than with either one alone. This combination of the two systems is called *autogenic feedback training*. Autogenic training supplies a strong, suggestive imagery and biofeedback supplies immediate knowledge of the results. These are powerful factors in gaining voluntary control of involuntary processes, and are of great importance in continuing research programs.

Many people in the medical profession are anxious to use any biofeedback techniques that will assist the patient in cooperating with the thera-

---

[11]Elmer Green & Alyce Green. (1973). The ins and outs of mind–body energy. *Science year, 1974: World book science annual.* Chicago: Field Enterprises Educational Corp., p. 138.
[12]Green & Green (1973), p. 141.

peutic program. Many in the medical profession now have biofeedback equipment in their offices. The goal, be it achieved with acupuncture or another method, is for the patient to be able to conduct self-therapy, leading to the healthiest life possible.

Alyce and Elmer Green at the Menninger Clinic in Topeka, Kansas, have developed a series of autogenic phrases that tend to bring the patient closer to the alpha brain wave rhythm. Particularly in situations when tension is a major part of the patient's problem, these phrases can be used by the one giving the massage to the patient,

> You feel quiet; you are beginning to feel quite relaxed; your feet feel heavy and relaxed; your ankles, your knees and your hips feel heavy, relaxed and comfortable; your solar plexus, and the whole central portion of your body, feel relaxed and quiet; your hands, your arms and your shoulders, feel heavy, relaxed and comfortable; your neck, your jaws and your forehead feel relaxed, they feel comfortable and smooth; your whole body feels quiet, heavy, comfortable and relaxed; you are quite relaxed; your arms and hands are heavy and warm; you feel quite quiet; your whole body is relaxed and your hands are warm, relaxed and warm; your hands are warm; warmth is flowing into your hands, they are warm, warm; you can feel the warmth flowing down your arms into your hands; your hands are warm, relaxed and warm; your whole body feels quiet, comfortable and relaxed; your mind is quiet; you withdraw your thoughts from the surroundings and you feel serene and still; your thoughts are turned inward and you are at ease; deep within your mind you can visualize and experience yourself as relaxed, comfortable, and still; you are alert, but in an easy, quiet, inward-turned way; your mind is calm and quiet; you feel an inward quietness.[13]

These phrases can be recorded on a cassette and given to the patient for home use.

It is a well-established fact that the patient's emotional reaction to pain must be resolved before pain can be relieved.

Melzack and the Greens have used alpha brain wave feedback training with patients suffering persistent pain.[14] Alpha brain rhythm is associated with feelings of calm. Experiments indicated that patients could relieve their pain by one third or more, and needed fewer analgesics following autogenic training.

## Use of Subliminal Messages in Healing

Recent developments in the field of subliminal psychology have led to the widespread use of prerecorded subliminal programs and guided imagery meditations. The Fenton River Center has combined these techniques into a

---

[13]Originally presented by Dr. Alyce Green at the Menninger Foundation, Topeka, Kan. Reprinted with permission.
[14]Ronald Melzack. (1973). *The puzzle of pain.* New York: Basic Books.

powerful process called "subliminally reinforced guided meditation."[15] The power of the subliminal message is that it is communicated directly to the nonconscious mind (subliminal meaning below the level of conscious awareness), thereby bypassing the judgmental, blocking process of the conscious, rational mind. This is done by encoding the message voices into the background sound or music just below the level of conscious perception. The listener hears only pleasant music, the ocean or other environmental sounds, or in the case of the "subliminally reinforced guided meditation" is guided through a focusing meditation by an audible guide voice while the subliminal messages are directed unnoticed to the nonconscious mind.

This particular program is based on the philosophy that all dis-ease is a result of misperception in the mind; that the natural state of existence is one of health and happiness, and that dis-ease is a projection of the fear, guilt, and anger accumulated since early childhood. The visualization procedures and subliminal messages in these meditations are designed to remove these blocks and stimulate the flow of natural healing forces. This allows the body to heal itself from within (where all true healing occurs) and to maintain a state of perfect health and emotional joy. The meditation is useful in preventative treatment as well as being a reinforcement for other types of healing.

In order to guard against taking on negative energy from the patient, therapists are cautioned not to recognize anything other than the potential state of perfect health. In addition to protecting themselves, therapists will be helping the patient to move toward a positive healing attitude. Focusing on the dis-ease can actually increase the problem by keeping the mind of the patient focused on the state of illness rather than the desired state of health. The meditation is most effective when practiced regularly by both the patient and the healer, and just prior to and during the treatment to open the healing channels. The healing power comes from the life force flowing through the patient and the healer, not from the healer's own energy. Actually, the healer benefits equally from this process.

Although the following meditation does not include the subliminal messages, it will enhance the healing massage. To prepare for the "Inner Light Meditation,"[16] relax and clear your mind. Use of a relaxation technique such as described in the previous section (Imagery and Subliminal Tapes) is helpful. The prerecorded "Inner Light Meditation" available from the Fenton River Center contains the relaxation instructions and the guided meditation as well as subliminal instructions for healing. It can be played during massage as well as any time thereafter in the privacy of the home to extend the healing power of the massage.

The following are excerpts from "Inner Light Meditation" and should

---

[15]Copyright by Fenton River Center, Storrs, Conn. Personal communication from Brian R. Ahern, M.S.W., Director (1987).

[16]Copyright by Fenton River Center, Storrs, Conn. Personal communication from Brian R. Ahern, M.S.W., Director (1987).

be spoken in a slow, steady, quiet, reassuring voice, allowing a full minute between each meditation:

1. Imagine a white light shining from deep within yourself; a beautiful, pure, radiant, bright light radiating outward. Feel the healing warmth of the light as it flows through you, surrounding you with a powerful protective aura.

2. Imagine a stream of light flowing from your internal source; flowing through you and out of your fingertips like a fountain of water, rising up into the air and falling back to the ground, splashing in a dazzling display of liquid light. Experience the refreshing healing power of the light as it washes back over you, soothing your body and mind of all discomfort.

3. With your mind, direct this stream of light to a destination of your choice. This may be a person or a group, a friend or an enemy, a nation or a world situation, or even a geological condition in the planet itself; anything or anyone which you feel needs the healing power of light. The light is infinite wisdom and infinite power. Trust the light to know the right and perfect means of its manifestation. All you need to do is guide the light to its destination. Do not try to determine just how it will work. You are the instrument of focusing and directing the light. The power and wisdom is in the light. Breathe deeply, relax. Feel the power and love and joy of the light as it flows through you. See the object of your meditation being filled with the healing power of light. The light is infinite power and the source of all creation. It can do anything.

4. Expand the light to surround the entire planet. See a cloud of pure, white, radiant light surrounding and filling everything on the surface of the planet. Feel the peace and power and love of the light as it flows through you.

## SUMMARY

The recent discovery of endorphins may soon provide answers to the neurophysiologic mechanisms involved in relief of pain by acupuncture or massage given to specific areas, such as Bindegewebsmassage. In addition, during massage the use of autogenic phrases will assist the patient to relax. Sensorimotor stimulation by massage facilitates the development of premature infants as well as decreasing the possibility of emotional disturbance.

# 7

# Reflections on the Choice of Method

Stephen Kitts, R.M.T.

Since ancient times, human beings have tried to help each others' ailments through some form of touch. Over time, these simple intuitive actions have been cultivated, studied, and organized into various systems and passed along through the generations. These systems were originally derived from empirical evidence, from "what worked." As they were transmitted through the ages, the systems acquired a certain body of theory to explain and support how they worked. Scientific research of the various forms of massage and body therapies has been sparse, whereas new information and techniques have been steadily increasing. With so many choices available, practitioners may wonder how to select the appropriate method or technique to use at any given time. A number of factors will be looked at while considering this question.

## TRAVEL, MAPS, AND TERRITORY

> *All training is a preparation to go beyond training. It is the effort we make to reach "the effortless."*
>
> —*Stephen Levine*[1]

Given a particular patient and condition to be addressed, in our considerations for the choice of method, one basic factor will be the practitioner's familiarity and skill with a potential system of massage therapy. For purposes of this study, it is assumed that the professional practitioner has at-

---

[1]Stephen Levine. (1982). *Who dies?* Garden City, NY: Anchor Press/Doubleday, p. 296.

**53**

tained the following as a basis for beginning practice and selecting a system:

1. Basic knowledge of anatomy, physiology, ethics, legalities, and hygiene relative to the safe and responsible performance of the work.
2. Knowledge of the system's theory, effects, indications, and contraindications.
3. Understanding of the importance of trust and openness in the healing relationship.
4. Practice and skill in applying techniques.

Beyond these basic considerations, the different systems of massage therapy could be regarded as maps abstracted from either an empirical or theoretical base. As the practitioner, what you experience in your travels—your sessions with individual patients—can be strongly influenced by the map you are following. A topographical map looks nothing like a road map and does not serve the same function. Furthermore, the maps may be excellent guides for relating to the same human territory, but the maps are not the actual experience of travelling. Actual hands-on work with people is a necessary part of learning the value of any particular system.

To continue the metaphor of travel, to begin the journey knowledge of the territory to be covered will be needed and a choice must be made between the various vehicles or methods for travel, each with its own map. Skill and understanding in the use of the vehicles or methods will also be required. Next, any preferences of vehicles will be considered and the destination or desired effect, with the current conditions for travel, must be known.

## CLIENT–THERAPIST PREFERENCES

> *Touching as a therapeutic event is not so simple as a mechanical procedure or a drug, because it is, above all, an act of communication. As in all embodied communication, the message being sent is not necessarily the same as the message received.*
>
> —*Ruth McCorkle, R.N., Ph.D.*
> *Margaret Hollenbach, Ph.D.*[2]

The therapist and patient both have a unique relationship with touch as a form of communication. Cultural and societal attitudes influence the style, the amount, and the circumstances that make touch acceptable and satisfying. These preferences can affect the way receivers experience and interpret

---

[2]Ruth McCorkle & Margaret Hollenbach. (1984). Touch and the acutely ill. In Catherine Caldwell Brown (Ed.), *The many faces of touch*. Skillman, NJ: Johnson & Johnson Baby Products Co., p. 176.

touch, and their ability to say how they want to be touched. From the practitioner's standpoint, these preferences can figure significantly in the choice of method. They may also have considerable impact on where one works, with whom, the quality of one's touch, and the openness with which it is received.

Certain attitudes on the part of the patient can have a very positive effect on massage therapy. The following description of helpful patient attitudes appears in a brochure from the Alternative Therapies Unit in San Francisco General Hospital.

> A good candidate for our program is a person who
>
> - acknowledges the existence of the problem and the possibility that life factors play a role;
> - is willing to work actively on it, i.e., to do "homework";
> - feels that s/he can take responsibility for and influence his state of health;
> - can connect experience with his body changes; sees the connection between what goes on in his mind and his body.
>
> People who do poorly in our program are
>
> - those who believe a pill or other "magic bullet" will solve the problem.[3]

Can practitioners' preferences ever hinder the healing process? Likes and dislikes may be subtle or deeply rooted habits in the mind. Certain preferences block creative moment-to-moment responses from flowing between client and therapist. A practitioner may prefer to massage or touch healthy people of the opposite sex. Touching a younger person may be preferred to touching or being touched by an elderly person. Someone may discover an aversion to holding or touching the sick, handicapped, or dying. A man may not be comfortable touching or being massaged by another man. Another person may show preference for massaging the well-defined muscles of body-builders and athletes. The same person may be averse to working with anyone overweight. Some practitioners feel they do not want to "deal with any emotional stuff." Barbara Roberts, R.N., C.M.T., observes that,

> it's like forms of artistic expression: Some artists love wood carving and dislike drawing; others love oil painting. Everyone is different. The body-workers who are the best are able to "read" intuitively their clients' needs, to perform quick physical assessment (integrating whatever medical information their clients give them), and to choose from a wide repertoire of styles or techniques that will particularly suit the needs of the client.[4]

---

[3]Alternative Therapies Unit, San Francisco General Hospital, San Francisco, CA.
[4]Barbara Roberts. (1984). *Physical assessment skills: A guide for the bodyworker.* Encinitas, CA: Author, p. 14.

When practitioner preferences exist, they can be conscious and communicated openly to patients, as in the following statement by Anne Patterson, an acupressure therapist and teacher from California:

> In my work and in my teaching, I emphasize gentleness and acceptance. I feel it is important to bring this approach into acupressure, (finger pressure to acupuncture points) a body therapy which is often feared and misunderstood as something which must hurt to have benefit. This is simply not true. Relaxation and change, be it physical or mental, cannot be forced. In the approach I take, the recipient has an active role to play in allowing the relaxation and health which the body instinctively seeks. The provider, although appearing the active one, actually assumes the major role of watching, encouraging, and trusting in the recipient's ability to allow the changes and seek the balance.[5]

## DESIRED EFFECT

Another consideration in choosing the method is the outcome desired. Before starting to work with someone, the practitioner meets with the patient. Information is shared that may include a previous medical diagnosis and prescription. If a prescription is given, the practitioner notes the type of treatment ordered, areas and structures of the body to be attended to, and prescribed frequency and duration of sessions. The prescription may also contain a plan for reevaluation with any additional comments or concerns. The practitioner listens attentively during this meeting, generally noting such factors as personality, body type, and other items that may arise from the history or questionnaire filled out by the patient.

Occasionally, a rather structured plan is designed based on what appears to be possible and acceptable to all concerned. A physician's diagnosis with prescription for massage may call for a specific physical effect. A person with residual muscle spasm from a prior accident may plan for a series of visits. A patient with limited movement and possible adhesions following an injury or surgery may seek relief in conjunction with other therapies.

At other times, the effect or outcome may be less defined. A person undergoing the stresses of a new job or a broken relationship may come in with "aches and pains all over." Anxieties at school or at home may bring someone with "that same old place in the back" starting to hurt again, wanting to explore habitual patterns and emotional issues in a conscious context of "safe touch." For some who are in chronic pain or dying, the presence, support, and touch in the moment-to-moment passage of time may be more the "purpose" than any hoped-for outcome.

People also come in for massage therapy when they just want to relax in a confidential, stress-free environment, with the desired effect being that of feeling "balanced . . . harmonized . . . whole." The practitioner may be

---

[5]Anne A. Patterson. (1980). *Acupressure workbook.* Unpublished manuscript. Berkeley, CA, p. 1.

given verbal or tacit permission to follow personal intuition, experiment, and otherwise *be there* to do whatever feels appropriate. With the amount of trust and spaciousness apparent in this relationship, the session encourages exploration and spontaneity. Specific goals or issues may or may not emerge during the session.

## EXISTING CONDITION

Many practitioners use a standard questionnaire with their patients. It is usually filled out at the time of the first visit. The questionnaire will ask for medical history in addition to personal information. It will gather data on any current symptom(s) the patient may have, and make available any information from a prior diagnosis, accident, injury, trauma, or surgery along with significant dates. Physical and psychologic determinations must be made to determine the appropriateness of a method as well as areas of the body where the work would be most beneficial.

During the time of information gathering, the practitioner considers a number of factors before actually doing any hands-on work. Even after beginning work on the patient, these concerns may be reassessed as needed. Considerations made before selecting any techniques or methods will generally include the following: (1) the patient's physical constitution and safety; (2) positioning concerns; (3) tissue density; (4) pressure and pain tolerance; (5) areas of specific emphasis and draping concerns; (6) the patient's size and age; (7) duration of session and apportionment of time; (8) need for lubricant or other equipment; (9) patient expectations and prior experience with massage therapy; and (10) any personal and cultural beliefs, attitudes, and preferences relating to the present condition and circumstances.

More information about the existing condition will appear when the patient is on the table. The practitioner may then use hands and fingers to detect much that on the surface appears hidden. Experienced hands have surprised many a massage patient with their ability to accurately locate "trouble spots" and relieve pain and tension stored there.

## CHOOSING

*Choosing may be only consenting to something that's happening at a semi-conscious level.*
—*Richard B. Clarke, Ph.D.*[6]

It seems there are two ways in which choices can occur. One way is the result of a rational process in which one gathers information, analyzes it, and makes a choice. Another way in which choices can occur is through an

---

[6]Richard B. Clarke. (1980, April). Workshop: The integration of psychotherapy and spiritual practice.

intuitive process whereby a direct knowledge or awareness *happens* without any conscious reasoning. When asked "How did you make that choice?" a practitioner may frequently reply, "I just know." A Zen teacher once said "You don't have to make the decision. Just become aware of the situation as it is, and the decision will be 'made'." Ongoing practice often cultivates a growing confidence in one's skills, along with a simultaneous trust in one's developing intuition.

Many practitioners follow a middle road with their patients. They collect information and make a mental plan or blueprint for the session(s) on the basis of the data received and an intuitive sense. This blueprint is held rather lightly, however, as the work actually begins. This is an acknowledgment of touch as a form of communication that is dynamic, direct, and capable of evoking a variety of unpredictable responses.

There are blueprints that suggest using only techniques from one system and evaluating the response after a few sessions. One practitioner may choose to use such a blueprint, whereas another may mix techniques from several systems in each session. One blueprint may work, another may not. Plans can change as necessary.

Beliefs about the importance of method choice vary considerably. A case can be made that it is not what one does that is important, but how one does it. Those who hold this belief can choose any method. The method does not matter, but whatever one chooses, one's skill and attitude should align with criteria established within the framework of that unique methodology. Some practitioners place equal importance on both what one does and how one does it. Therefore, a careful decision is necessary both in choosing appropriate techniques and in applying them with correct attitude and competency. Another belief is that it is neither what one does nor how one does it that matters, as it is the patient or receiver who heals himself or herself; the practitioner is only a channel. Beyond this belief lies the question "Who does what to whom?"

Choice can therefore include many possibilities. As Jules Older notes, "As with so many forms of healing, individual responses differ so markedly that generalization is almost impossible."[7] Ultimately, people choose and act with the information, skills, and consciousness of the moment. Choosing or aligning with the path of least harm and most heart, they do their best, and they can accept the outcome without any special attachment to the results.

As Andrew Weil concludes, "The existence and success of therapeutic systems based on mutually inconsistent theories and methods must be accounted for by any general theory of health and healing. It suggests that factors other than theories and methods determine whether medical interventions succeed or fail."[8]

---

[7]Jules Older. (1982). *Touching is healing*. Briarcliff Manor, NY: Stein & Day, p. 233.
[8]Andrew Weil. (1983). *Health and healing*. Boston: Houghton Mifflin, p. 194.

## Specific Examples

The following cases have been included to illustrate possible choices that can be made using combinations of techniques from three popular systems, namely Swedish massage, Shiatsu (a system using direct pressure over acupuncture points, passive stretches, and joint movements, described in Chapter 22), and Polarity (a system of gentle touching to release energy blocks, described in Chapter 23). There are also some additional considerations given for each of the sample cases and conditions. One intention in showing sample cases is to indicate how well different methods can integrate with one another. The cases are also offered as pointers for expanding the number of choices and possibilities for practice. They are meant to encourage exploration in the application of methods. The cases are not meant to offer stock formulas, as there is no way of knowing how to respond until one is actually present with the client.

### CASE 1: GENERAL FATIGUE

A 37-year-old woman complains of fatigue and irritability since the recent holiday season. She feels that she has been caring for everyone's needs but her own, and now she wants to give herself a gift of relaxing massage.

**Possible Session**

*Swedish massage:* give general relaxing Swedish massage with special attention to areas of tension. *Polarity:* intersperse Polarity techniques with Swedish massage for stimulating parasympathetic nervous system, thus deepening the state of relaxation. *Shiatsu:* work feet and hands.

**Additional Considerations**

Each of our three sample systems has elements that can help bring forth the most relaxed response to the work. In Swedish massage, the tempo and rhythm of stroking and kneading often add to the comfort and relaxation of the patient. In the same way, the Polarity practitioner may use rhythmical oscillations and gentle holding. The Shiatsu practitioner may seek a rhythm harmonizing the pressure and release with the breathing of the receiver.

The voice tone of the practitioner may convey certain feelings of warmth and relaxation. There may be a selection of music from which the receiver may choose a piece of special background music. Environmental elements such as heat, lighting, and ventilation should all be checked before starting the session. Be prepared for the possibility that massage may free the patient to express previously suppressed emotions, for this is a common response and may be as therapeutic as the bodywork itself.

### CASE 2: AN OLDER CLIENT

A 65-year-old man has chronic low back pain, secondary to chronic postural strain and poor body mechanics. He has been cleared by both a chiropractor and a medical doctor.

**Possible Session**

*Shiatsu:* give massage to paravertebral muscles (bladder meridians), buttocks, and legs. *Polarity:* use low amplitude oscillations at the beginning of range of motion over transverse processes of the vertebrae, gently rocking the entire body to encourage muscular relaxation and increased segmental mobility of vertebrae. *Swedish massage:* use effleurage, petrissage, and deep friction over paraspinal muscles.

### Additional Considerations

A shorter session is often advisable for older people, particularly in beginning work, so as not to overtax them. An elderly person may be uncomfortable lying too long in any one position, or may find it difficult to turn over or raise or lower himself or herself. It may be difficult for older patients to lower themselves onto the floor for Shiatsu, for example. Extra support may also be needed for increased comfort due to physical changes from aging, posture, surgery, etc. Some elderly patients chill easily and may require a warmer room temperature or perhaps a flannel blanket or heating pad. If practicing massage or Polarity on a standard-sized table, it may be good to have a small step-stool available for older patients' ease in climbing onto the table.

When performing massage, be mindful of older patients' drier, less elastic skin and thinner tissues, requiring less force or pressure. If using any oil on the feet, it is best to remove it thoroughly to eliminate any chance that patients might slip and fall when they are back home, in their bathrooms, for instance. Allow enough time for changing clothes since elderly patients may have on several layers of clothing, may require assistance, or may move rather slowly. They may also enjoy talking with you as much as the massage or touch.

### CASE 3: TERMINAL ILLNESS

A 58-year-old woman is dying of cancer. Doctors say she has only a few weeks to live. Her husband has asked you to come and perhaps help relieve some of the anxiety and tension that prevent her from sleeping now.

### Possible Session

*Swedish massage:* give light massage to face and hands. *Shiatsu:* work on area around eyes, posterior neck and occiput, feet. *Polarity:* rest one hand (or hold above body) at level of belly while the other rests on or above the heart. Next move one hand to the area on or above the heart, and the other on or above the forehead. Remove hands very gently.

### Additional Considerations

Stay present and just *be* with the person. It is most likely that you will be entering their space where bed, supports, comforts, etc. have already been in use. Enter gently, respond mindfully and heartfully. Stephen Levine, a writer, teacher of meditation, and counselor for the terminally ill, offers the following general considerations for those providing care to the dying.

> Comfort is the primary goal of physical care. Give the individual what he needs as often as he needs it without projecting any need of your own. Be flexible; no rules, just be tuned to the moment and trust your own heart's sense of what is appropriate. Unless asked, the fewer opinions the better, of how one should die. Just allow that being his own process. Be sensitive to the constantly changing condition of the individual. Sometimes someone might want to be held or massaged. At another moment only medication will be sufficient. One needs to be sensitive to another and to oneself so that one's own fear does not close around one.[9]

---

[9]Levine (1982), p. 296.

Barbara Blattner, R.N., M.P.H., author of *Holistic Nursing*, gives a very personal account of massaging the feet of a dying friend.

I wanted to give everything. Everything that was possible in the whole world to a thirty-one-year-old friend, dying of cancer who merely had the strength to lie in a hospital bed and look out at the San Francisco skyline and the hills of Sausalito.

How much can you feel through your feet? I looked up at Stef's face and wondered if I should stop, if this was too exhausting. I wanted to go on. He's only partly here, I thought. He comes and he goes, back and forth from this world to the next. I don't like letting go of him but there's no choice. This is the only way that he can experience this massage—on his terms, not on mine.

I stayed with his feet as he dozed. In a short while, he came back and opened his eyes again. I was relieved to see him and know that he was still here. I kept going until I felt finished. I capped his foot with my hands and wrapped it back up beneath the blankets.

I felt complete and full and satisfied. But I was surprised that instead of feeling like falling apart, I felt calm and peaceful.

There was no fear—there was simply being. Stefan was being exactly where he was—partly here and partly there. And he let me into the space beneath the covers.[10]

## CASE 4: LABOR AND DELIVERY

A 31-year-old woman has asked for her massage therapist to be present during her labor and delivery.

### Possible Session
*Shiatsu:* give pressure to low back and buttocks, and Spleen 6. *Polarity:* connect uterus points on inner ankle with lower abdomen, front to back hand contacts over lower abdomen and belly, or light perineal contact with right hand, left hand on back of neck. *Swedish massage:* use light effleurage from proximal to distal along inner legs, with light circular movements over abdomen.

### Additional Considerations
Once labor begins, be aware that the mother's emotional and physical state will be changing rapidly. For example, even if the mother has been planning on receiving massage therapy during labor, she may decide she does not want to be touched when the actual time arrives. Certain points may prove to be more effective than others in stimulating contractions, focusing the mother's attention, or reducing pain, and the points themselves may change as the labor progresses. Let the mother guide you, and avoid bothering her with too many questions.

Some find that stimulation of the uterus point on the inner ankle is effective in stimulating contractions, others find it slows them down. If back labor is present, the mother may prefer direct strong stimulation over the low back and sacral area. The mother's position will often limit choices and her choice for positioning should come before any need of the massage practitioner.

During pushing, with the mother sitting and leaning back against pillows or the husband, light effleurage may be done on the inner legs from belly to feet, repeating "down and out" while keeping eye contact.

Another possibility is a Polarity and Swedish massage combination, with the therapist seated at the mother's left side while she is sitting up. Put the right

---

[10]Barbara Blattner. (1981). *Holistic nursing.* Englewood Cliffs, NJ: Prentice Hall, pp. 441–442.

hand behind her back and the left hand over her belly. Do coordinated "round and rounds" of *very* light effleurage. (If the labor is long, use a *lot* of oil and work lightly, not with direct pressure, so the effleurage does not irritate the skin.)

The following suggestions come from the book *Massage and Peaceful Pregnancy* by Gordon Inkeles.

> When it works, massage during labor or delivery requires more endurance than fancy technique from the masseur. Usually a woman will ask you to concentrate on one or two parts of her body—say, the shoulders and lower back. She may have a favorite movement, such as shoulder friction, to which you can add occasional hand-over-hand stroking, fingertip kneading, and circulation movements for variation. Be ready to continue for the better part of an hour if necessary. If you become fatigued, see if somebody else can take over while you rest. Team massage works well during labor because less experienced members of the team need learn only a few strokes to be effective. Choose calm people for your team who will be content to copy a few basic movements without improvising.[11]

## CASE 5: PATIENT WITH SCHIZOPHRENIA

A 22-year-old man who has experienced periodic schizophrenic episodes wants to feel more "connected with his body." With the supervision of his psychiatrist, this patient is coming to you for his first experience of massage therapy.

### Possible Session
*Swedish massage:* give an abbreviated general massage (30 to 35 min). *Shiatsu:* back and buttocks along bladder meridian, feet, and hands. *Polarity:* is not recommended as treatment of choice for beginning work. One or two manipulations may be done and response evaluated.

### Additional Considerations
This first visit is shortened a bit to allow extra time for evaluating the patient's response and to prevent overtaxing him or her. The practitioner should be alert to the patient's breathing during the session, helping the receiver "ground" awareness in his or her body through somewhat slower movements, eye contact, and verbal communication as needed. Rapport and patient perception of safety could be considered of central importance in this session. Any form of traction is not recommended. Swedish massage, Shiatsu, and Polarity all have a variety of techniques that can be learned for home use.

Used sensitively, massage may be a helpful adjunct to psychotherapeutic care. Older notes that there are many ways in which massage can soothe the psyche as well as the body.

> What does go on in healing massage? I think there are several components. The most important is legitimized skin-to-skin contact in a safe situation. . . .
>
> A second component is the masseuse's acceptance of the client's problems and pain combined with a readiness to treat them actively. . . .
>
> Another factor is direct, caring attention to hurt parts of the body, parts that often have direct links to hurt feelings. Attending to a sore shoulder can release feelings about aging; massaging a disabled leg can bring out feelings about deformity. Thus can massage connect mind and body, or, perhaps more correctly, close the imagined gap between them. . . .

---

[11]Gordon Inkeles. (1983). *Massage and peaceful pregnancy.* New York: Putnam, p. 122.

Finally there is the expectation of positive results, an aid to almost any form of healing, and in massage, a natural result of the combination of other components.

These elements transcend beliefs about polarity, ch'i energy, acupressure, chiropractic, or osteopathy. If they are present, the client is likely to arise from the table feeling warm, open, relaxed, and invigorated. If they are not, forget it.[12]

The previous five cases demonstrate the facility with which a well-trained massage practitioner can draw from various types of massage. Of course, these are just examples and no one sequence can be the "right" one. One patient may respond better to deeper work, another to lighter work, regardless of the nature of the problem. The well-trained massage practitioner has a minimum of 500 hours of supervised in-class instruction and thus can respond with a wide variety of techniques in an appropriate manner.

## SUMMARY

What is "healing" after all? Dr Weil points out the limits to an intellectual approach to health care.

Every system I have examined fails to work some of the time, regardless of how logical and scientifically sound its theory, how careful its application, and how strong its indication for a particular problem or patient. Again, the frequency of failures is not known, but in my experience it is considerable for all systems, allopathy included.

The question of why treatments fail, when theory and experience predict success, is as important as the question of why treatments work when science can demonstrate their theories to be fallacious.[13]

Questions and confusions may continue to surface for the practitioner. True questioning can serve us by deepening our training, practice, and trust, challenging practitioners to let go and embrace unknowns; to give and not close themselves to receiving; to act and go on with arms open wide. For the patient as well, questions and concerns may continue to arise. In the introduction to his book *Awakening the Heart*, John Welwood speaks to these concerns for the benefit of all patients and therapists, and the patient–therapist in all of us.

First of all, it is important to recognize that the therapeutic encounter, like any intimate relationship, is full of mystery, surprise, and unpredictable turns. No matter how well trained therapists are in psychological theory and therapeutic technique, the encounter with another human being who seeks relief from suffering invariably challenges them in ways that their

---

[12]Older (1982), p. 101.
[13]Weil (1983), p. 194.

clinical training has not prepared them for. Most therapists will admit, at least privately, that they often do not know just what is going on for their clients, that they are often uncertain and at a loss about how to help their clients. If a therapist perceives this uncertainty as a threat to his expertise, then he might treat it as a sign of failure or defeat. But when healing is seen as a mutual opportunity for real opening, a therapist can approach these moments of uncertainty in a different way. For they do challenge the therapist to put aside his theories and beliefs for the moment, and to pay closer attention both to the client and to his own responses in order to get a better sense for what is happening. These moments of uncertainty, when the therapist has to let go of his mental agenda, may force him into a more direct relationship with the client. At these times, a new quality of sharpened perception and "being with" the client can emerge if the therapist does not fall back on theory and technique when he does not know what to do next. As the therapist's need to be in control relaxes, he can be present with more heart.[14]

---

[14]John Welwood. (1983). *Awakening the heart*. Boston & London: New Library, Shambala, p. ix.

# PART II

# The Application of Basic Western Techniques

# 8

# General Procedures of Massage

## BEGIN CAUTIOUSLY

Generally, massage begins with light effleurage that follows the venous flow. Do not massage directly over the most tender areas or the actual site of injury, but proximal to it. As the patient grows accustomed to the touch, the involved area can then be cautiously approached. When the patient can tolerate rather deep effleurage one may work into petrissage. This may be light or deep depending again on the extent of the involvement and tolerance of the patient.

If other techniques such as friction, cross-fiber manipulation, and tapotement are used, they follow the use of effleurage and petrissage. Effleurage is usually interspersed with other strokes and is the stroke ordinarily used to begin and finish a massage treatment.

In concluding the treatment, strokes that work gradually from deep to light should be used. If used at all, tapotement is most often given at the end of the massage treatment as a terminal touch. It is not normally used in therapeutic situations unless on stump ends. It is often used in athletic situations or for other stimulation.

## USE ORIGINALITY

Judgment and originality must be used to find the correct approach with each patient. In many cases that which "feels good" will be a strong factor in choice of strokes. At other times whether it feels good or not, certain techniques will be necessary. Each stroke has a purpose. It becomes the responsibility of the operator to judge from the tissues beneath the working hands which techniques to select, how deep the pressure should be, how gentle the stretching must be, when to progress from one stroke to another, and when to progress from one area to another.

It is never wise to spend too long in one small area. It is more advisable to massage the whole general area, coming back to the areas of tenderness often.

## KNOW THE OBJECTIVES

The objective of each treatment should be kept in mind. Each case will have one or more problems, such as pain, limited motion, swelling, etc., that require special attention.

If massage is given for a sedative purpose, the strokes will be slow and rhythmical, using effleurage and petrissage with pressure that is not too deep. Slow, rhythmical effleurage with the part in elevation will reduce edema. If the desired effect is stimulation, the speed of the stroke can be increased and deeper pressure can be used.

## FOLLOW MUSCLE GROUPS

The operator needs to be aware of the muscle groups involved in each case. The usual procedure is to massage each muscle group (for example the flexors of a joint), applying effleurage and petrissage that can be followed by friction or any other special strokes that may seem indicated. Each muscle group should be "stroked off" with effleurage before proceeding to the next muscle group.

There are times when one may need to approach the involved part by some division other than by muscle groups. The operator may massage the anterior aspect of the body before approaching the posterior in order to avoid asking the patient to turn over more than once. In so doing, the operator should still be aware of the muscle or muscle group that is being massaged.

When muscular tightness is present, friction to the tendons, toward their insertion, will help relieve protective muscle splinting against pain.

## SUMMARY

Aside from these general remarks, it is not the feeling of this author that specific instruction can be given for any specific involvement. The operator must be aware of the basic conditions that exist, such as pain, swelling, limited motion, etc., and treat these symptoms, regardless of whether they are caused by surgery, accident, or illness. After learning to apply massage techniques to the various areas of the body, the student will be ready to study the cases in Part V to learn how to plan individual routines for specific situations.

# 9

# Effleurage

Effleurage is used more than any other of the massage techniques. It usually initiates each treatment. The evaluation the operator can make of the patient's soft tissue with this technique can be a better orientation than a written or verbal report. During these initial strokes, sensitive fingers can explore for areas of tenderness or tightness. Effleurage is often interspersed between other strokes; it is used to progress from one area to another, and is the most common stroke used in concluding the treatment. Thus, it should be mastered, so that it can be performed with rhythm and confidence.

Any stroke that glides over the skin without attempting to move the deep muscle masses is called effleurage. The hand is molded to the part, stroking with firm and even pressure, usually upward.

## PURPOSE OF EFFLEURAGE

This stroke is usually used at the beginning and end of every massage as well as between all other strokes. It accustoms the patient to the touch of the operator and allows sensitive fingers to search for areas of spasm and soreness. In given instances where extreme soreness is present, it may be the only stroke employed. It serves to distribute evenly whatever lubricant is being used. Deep effleurage will also provide a passive stretch to given muscles or muscle groups. The muscles of the back are illustrated in Figure 9-1.

**69**

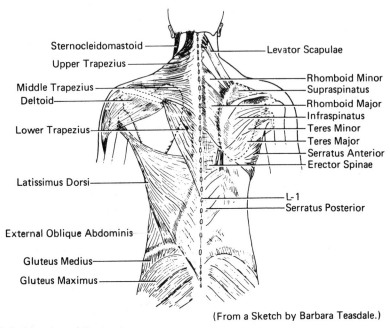

Sternocleidomastoid
Upper Trapezius
Middle Trapezius
Deltoid
Lower Trapezius
Latissimus Dorsi
External Oblique Abdominis
Gluteus Medius
Gluteus Maximus

Levator Scapulae
Rhomboid Minor
Supraspinatus
Rhomboid Major
Infraspinatus
Teres Minor
Teres Major
Serratus Anterior
Erector Spinae
L-1
Serratus Posterior

(From a Sketch by Barbara Teasdale.)

**Figure 9-1.** Muscles of the back.

## EFFLEURAGE TO THE BACK

### Position

First see that the patient is comfortable, lying prone with the feet either off the end of the treatment table or supported at the ankle by a roll or pillow. A pillow under the abdomen is often a good idea and the arms may be placed wherever they are most comfortable. The head may be turned to either side.

In cases when it is difficult for a patient to lie down and rise, treatment can be conducted in a sitting position. If this is done, the arms and head can be rested against the treatment table and supported by pillows, if necessary. Naturally, the patient must be seated on a stool or sideways on a chair so that the back can be free for treatment.

### Draping

The patient is asked to loosen or remove any clothing that might interfere with the massage. This can be done after the patient has been covered with a sheet. If assistance is needed, it should be given when asked for, or if the operator notices that it is needed. It is usually easier for the patient to loosen all clothing before turning to lie prone. The operator then pulls the sheet down to the level of the coccyx, being careful not to expose the gluteal cleft. The sheet can be tucked over the edge of the patient's clothing or pajamas in order to protect them from the lubricant. This draping will suffice for these early practice techniques. If the low back is involved the entire gluteal area should be massaged. This is discussed more thoroughly in Chapter 14.

## Application

Since powder leaves a clear pattern to follow, apply it using enough so a pattern can be seen when learning this stroke. Remember that too much powder will prevent good contact between the hand and the skin. Place both hands on the patient's back at the level of the coccyx, with the heel of the hand close to the spine and the fingers pointing outward. Make sure the whole hand is relaxed so that the entire palmar surface touches the patient's body. Allow the hands to glide slowly along the erector spinae group, being careful to avoid the spinous processes. As the neck is approached, the hands move upward to the base of the skull.

The return stroke downward may have lighter pressure progressing laterally, with the fingers molding over and in front of the shoulder to encompass the whole upper trapezius. As the stroke progresses, it follows the fibers of the upper trapezius to the shoulders and thence down the latissimus dorsi to the upper half of the gluteals (Fig. 9–2).

Effleurage may be light or deep depending on the amount of pressure applied, but this pressure should be the same throughout the stroke, until the student learns more about how to vary it.

### Points to Check While Practicing

1. Is the patient *comfortable?*
2. Is the patient *relaxed?*
3. Are the *hands* of the operator relaxed?

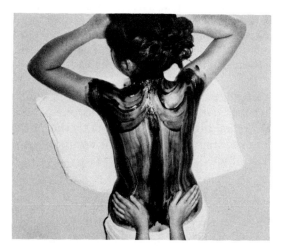

**Figure 9–2.** Fingerpaint pattern of effleurage.

4. Is pressure *even* throughout each stroke?
5. Is the stance one of good body alignment, with weight over feet, or has the weight been allowed to fall forward over the treatment table?
6. Is *all* of the hand in contact with the patient?
7. Look at the powder patterns on the patient's back. Compare them with Figure 9–2.

## VARIATIONS OF EFFLEURAGE

Whenever the pressure of any effleurage stroke over any part of the body is light, it is referred to as *light effleurage* regardless of the part of the body to which it is applied or the pattern that may be followed.

By the same token, any effleurage wherein the pressure is deep is referred to as *deep effleurage*. Stroking and effleurage are terms that may be used synonymously.

The student should attempt to maintain light pressure throughout the entire stroke and again deep pressure for the whole stroke. If this is done well, the student may then try to begin applying pressure lightly and increase until the pressure is quite deep, tapering off again until it is quite light at the end of the stroke. The student should then ask the patient to act as a guide by telling the student which pressure feels best, remembering that this "patient" is not one with an injured or arthritic back, but an essentially healthy one.

**Knuckling** is a stroke particularly associated with the techniques of Hoffa. In describing it he says,

> If the part to be treated is covered by thick fascia, effleurage is not deep enough. You need greater pressure, therefore the convex dorsal sides of the first interphalangeal joints must be used. Clench the fist in strong palmar flexion; the peripheral end of the knuckles should be upwards. Gradually bring the hand from plantar to dorsal flexion. Pressure is not continuous, but swells up and down, starting lightly and becoming stronger, then decreasing again in pressure. The hand must not adhere to the part but should glide over it lightly. Knuckling should only be used where there is enough room for the hand to be applied (*see* Fig. 9–3).[1]

**Shingles** refers to an alternate type of stroking in which one hand follows the other with the strokes overlaying themselves one after the other like the shingles on a roof. Thus, although contact with the patient is lost as each hand is lifted, the remaining hand maintains contact, giving the patient a feeling of constant contact.

---

[1]Albert J. Hoffa. (1978). *Technik der massage* (14th ed.). (Ruth Friedlander, Trans.) Stuttgart: Ferdinand Enke, p. 2.

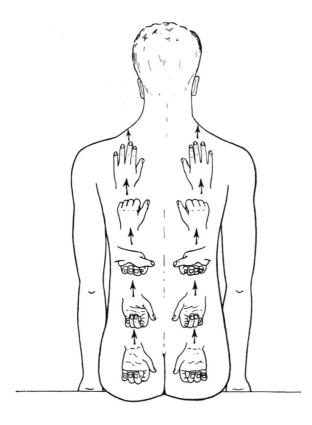

**Figure 9-3.** Application of knuckling stroke.

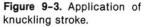

**Bilateral tree stroking** refers to both hands progressing simultaneously on either side of the back, from the spine laterally, and upward with short strokes that build like the branches growing from the trunk of a tree.

**Three-count stroking of the trapezius** (Fig. 9–4) can be done with a rhythmical three-count stroke that begins at the origin of the lower trapezius, progressing with one hand toward the insertion. Simultaneously, the other hand moves to the origin of the middle trapezius where it begins its stroke just as the first hand concludes, progressing toward the insertion of the middle trapezius. As soon as the first hand has completed its stroke of the lower trapezius, it progresses *without contact* to the origin of the upper trapezius and strokes downward to the insertion to complete the third part of this three-count routine. This particular method of stroking the whole trapezius is rhythmical and relaxing when well done, but it must be timed like the shingles strokes so that, in spite of the lost contact, as each hand is raised, the patient feels constant contact because one hand is always stroking.

**Horizontal stroking** is particularly useful when applied to the low back. Place both hands lightly on the patient's back as shown in Figure 9–5. Using a stroke similar to effleurage, move the right hand forward and the left hand backward with firm pressure. When the hands have gone as far to

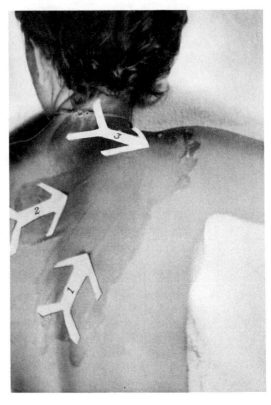

**Figure 9-4.** Three-count stroking of the trapezius.

the sides of the patient as possible, the stroke direction is reversed *without* changing the position of the hands. As the hands return to their original position a strong *lift* and *push together* of the hips is executed. The returning hands continue all the way over to the opposite side of the patient, thus going from side to side across the back. No pressure should be placed over the spinous processes as the hands pass over them. Greatest pressure comes into the *lift* and *push together* of the low back as the hands pull upward and inward to meet and cross over the spinous processes and continue on down each side of the patient. This feels especially good to the patient who has a sacroiliac involvement.

**Mennell's superficial stroking** can be distinguished from light effleurage by its unidirectional flow "going either centripetally or centrifugally but never in both directions," and by its return stroke through the air which must be "controlled as for rhythm" taking as long as that part of the stroke which contacts the patient. Only the lightest possible pressure is used in this stroke.[2]

---

[2]James B. Mennell. (1945). *Physical treatment by movement, manipulation and massage* (5th ed.). Philadelphia: Blakiston's Son, pp. 24–27.

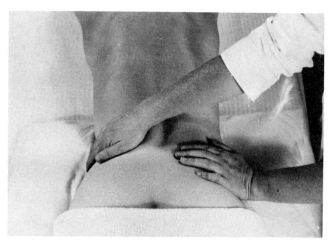

**Figure 9-5.** Horizontal stroking to the low back.

**Concluding stroke for relaxation** is used if preparing the patient to relax for sleep. The treatment is concluded with long, light, effleurage strokes that start at the base of the skull, stroking directly over the spinous processes, going all the way down to the coccyx. Pressure must be very light but firm and the rhythm monotonous; pressure that is too light would stimulate rather than sedate. As one hand is about to complete the stroke near the coccyx, the other hand begins the next stroke starting at the base of the skull, giving the patient the feeling of continuous contact, with one hand beginning the next stroke before the other finishes. If this technique is kept up for a minute or two it helps the patient relax completely. The patient often obtains a tingling sensation throughout the arms and legs that facilitates relaxation. Some patients will even fall asleep before the treatment is finished. If this technique is applied beyond two or three minutes, it tends to stimulate rather than relax so it should never be continued for long.

## SUMMARY

The effleurage strokes most often used in America today have been discussed. They should not limit the creative person who wishes to develop other types of effleurage strokes to suit the individual needs of a patient. Neither should the operator be restricted in adjusting the strokes described here on the back to all other parts of the body. The study of petrissage will teach the student how to combine these two massage techniques. While learning petrissage, effleurage should be interspersed between petrissage strokes for two reasons: to provide practice for the student, and to prevent "over petrissage" on any part of the body.

# —10——

# Petrissage

Petrissage is difficult to describe, but not difficult to perform. Contrary to effleurage, which glides over the skin, petrissage strokes attempt to lift the muscle mass and wring or squeeze it gently. Care should be taken not to work in one area too long before progressing to the next and not to pinch or bruise the tissues. These strokes should be practiced on the back until they can be done rhythmically and with good close contact before attempted on other parts of the body.

Petrissage consists of kneading manipulations that press and roll the muscles under the hands. It can be done with one hand, where the area to be kneaded is small, or it can be done with two hands on larger areas. It can even be done with two fingers on very small areas. There is no gliding over the skin except between progressions from one area to another.

## PURPOSE OF PETRISSAGE

This kneading motion of petrissage serves to "milk" the muscle of waste products that collect due to abnormal inactivity. It assists the venous return and in given instances it will also help to free adhesions.

Position and draping for application of petrissage to the back would be the same as that for effleurage (*see* Chapter 9).

## TWO-HAND PETRISSAGE TO THE BACK

Because all petrissage is preceded by effleurage as a preliminary stroke, review the effleurage strokes, first stroking lightly and then working gradually into a deep effleurage.

Now place both hands firmly on one side of the patient's back, with the lower hand ready to start in motion over the upper portion of the gluteals.

Although each hand is going to describe a circle, counterclockwise in direction, they do so with such timing that as one hand moves away from the spine across the muscles of the back, the other hand is moving medially toward the spine (Fig. 10–1). The hands are almost *flat* as they shape themselves to the contours of the back. They pick the tissues up *between* the hands (not *with* the hands), and as they "pass" each other the forceful part of the stroke is executed as the muscles are pressed downward against the ribs and rolled between the hands.

After about three repetitions of this stroke in one position, progress upward by allowing the lower hand to slide up to where the top hand has just been working, as the top hand glides upward to a new position.

Petrissage does not require much lubricant. The hands should cling to the part being massaged, picking up and pressing, sliding only when progressing, and even then with enough pressure so that fluids in the tissues are carried along with the stroke.

## VARIATIONS OF PETRISSAGE

### Alternating Two-Hand Petrissage to the Back

This type of petrissage for the back is very useful for following the direction of muscle fibers such as the trapezius.

Alternately use the index and middle fingers of one hand working with the thumb of the other hand. The thumbs are placed one above the other (Fig. 10–2) and remain in this position, although the emphasis of each stroke is carried first by one hand and then the other. The fingers of one hand reach proximally, pick up the muscle, and move toward the opposite thumb. At the same time, the thumb is pressing toward the proximal aspect of the muscle, moving toward the fingers. The opposite hand then repeats this same motion, and both hands alternately work from distal to proximal aspects of the muscle group.

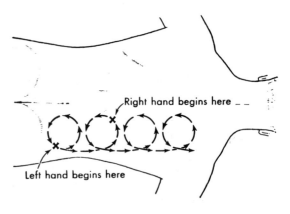

Right hand begins here

Left hand begins here

**Figure 10-1.** Petrissage of the back.

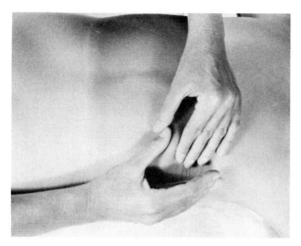

**Figure 10-2.** Alternating two-hand petrissage to the back.

## Two-Finger Petrissage on Broad Flat Areas

Following the erector spinae muscle group up the back, grasp a small part between the thumb and first finger. Press it out as is done in other petrissage strokes. Although the movement is small, the whole motion should come through a relaxed arm.

Other variations of petrissage are best practiced on areas smaller to grasp. Positioning and draping are described in Chapter 14 with the discussion of massage to the upper extremity. For purposes of this early practice they can be referred to briefly.

When applying any of the following techniques to areas of the body other than the back, "C" and "V" positions of the hand are used.

The C and V position names are derived from the C-like formation of the hand position as it grasps the arm or leg with the thumb in abduction and slightly flexed with the fingers cupped to fit the part being massaged. Pressure is exerted on the palm and the palmar surface of all fingers according to the contour of the part (Figs. 10–3, 10–4). The wide or open C would be applied to the hand position where a large area such as the thigh is involved (Fig. 10–3). The narrow, or closed C (Figs. 10–4, 10–5) refers to the use of the same position when it is applied to an arm or smaller area. On very narrow areas the position is so narrowed that the thumb comes into adduction and the position is then referred to as the V position (Fig. 10–6).

## One-Hand Petrissage

For use on smaller limbs (arms and children's legs) one hand is sufficient for petrissage. Place the hand *around* the part, picking up the muscle mass, using the *whole* hand. Lift the muscle away from the bone, squeezing gently upward and making small circular motions. Let the hand relax on the downward part of this small circle.

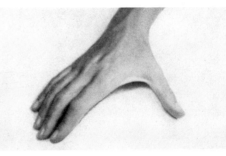

**Figure 10-3.** Open C position.

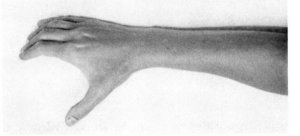

**Figure 10-4.** Closed C position.

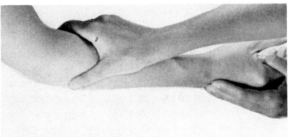

**Figure 10-5.** Closed C position.

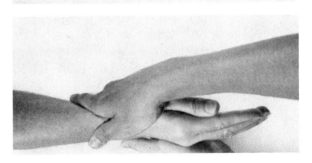

**Figure 10-6.** V position.

As with the two-hand petrissage, the rhythm should be slow and regular. Progression upward to a new position should follow three or four strokes. As the hand progresses, pressure is upward, carrying the venous return and lymph with it.

Since the biceps offers a distinctive, easily grasped muscle, apply one-hand petrissage to the upper arm. Let the muscle belly fit into the palm of the hand while the thumb and fingers apply pressure to the upward part of the stroke.

### Alternate One-Hand Petrissage

Another approach to petrissage of the upper arm may be accomplished by grasping the biceps in one hand and the triceps in the other. Using an alternate pattern of squeezing, petrissage both the flexors and the extensors with a soothing rhythm. As the one hand is relaxed, the other is putting on pressure with the same, upward, circular strokes.

In circumstances where a certain amount of stimulation is indicated, this stroke can be used to advantage, progressing rather rapidly with each stroke working always in the direction of the venous flow.

### SUMMARY

Other variations of petrissage are included in Part IV. These fine differences should not be attempted until the basic approach has been mastered. Later, if the operator can perform one technique better than the other, the preferred technique can be selected. While learning friction, both effleurage and petrissage should be interspersed, as people practicing on each other often work too deeply and bruise the tissues.

# ——11——
# Friction

Although massage could consist of only effleurage and petrissage, friction is necessary to reach beneath the more superficial tissues. Storms and Cyriax think that friction is the most important massage technique and base most of their massage treatment around this stroke.[1] When used correctly, it permits the operator to work into the deeper tissues gradually, judging how far to go by the patient's reaction.

Friction is performed by small circular movements with the tips of the fingers, the thumb, or the heel of the hand, according to the area to be covered. Small flat ellipsoids are described that penetrate into the depth of the tissue, not by moving the fingers on the *skin* but by moving the tissues *under* the skin.

## PURPOSE OF FRICTION

Friction is used to massage deep into the joint spaces or around bony prominences such as the patella. It is especially useful around a well-healed scar to break down adhesions between the skin and tissues beneath it. It *cannot* affect a deep fibrositis such as might form within a muscle belly.

## APPLICATION OF FRICTION TO THE BACK

Arrange the patient as for a back massage and begin the treatment with effleurage and then petrissage.

---

[1]Harold Storms. (1944, September). Diagnostic and therapeutic massage. *Archives of Physical Medicine, XXV,* 550.

Using the ball of each thumb, place one on each side of the spinous process of the back (Fig. 11–1). Any level of the back will do for a spot to learn the technique. Press as deeply as the patient can tolerate without pain, describing small circles with a force that comes down through the arm from the shoulder. These small circles do not slide across the skin (as effleurage does), nor do they "pick up" or "squeeze" (as petrissage does). They gradually press into the tissues, becoming deeper as the patient develops tolerance to the pressure. Pressure should never be released suddenly.

Progress upward after about three cycles, following bilaterally upward to the side of the spinous processes, and in the muscular spaces between the transverse processes. The student learning friction should never practice too long in one spot because attempts to obtain deep pressure may cause bruising until his or her own strength is learned and the technique adjusted accordingly.

Pressure continues up either side of the spine, avoiding the bony prominences. Following deep friction, effleurage stroking of the immediate area may be done with the thumbs to help the patient relax.

While the thumbs are doing the major portion of the work with this technique, the rest of the hand rests lightly on the back. It does not brace the thumb.

## VARIATIONS OF FRICTION

### Cross-Fiber Manipulation

Deep friction-like strokes that apply pressure *across* the muscle fiber rather than along the longitudinal axis of the muscle fibers can be applied to the erector spinae group of the back. Unlike typical friction strokes, the thumb moves across the skin with deep short strokes.

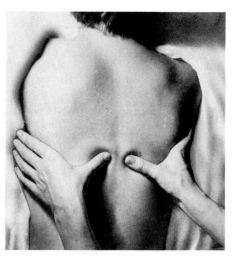

**Figure 11–1.** Friction.

Place one thumb close to the spinous process and stroke outward with deep pressure. Follow this stroke immediately by repeating the action with the other thumb, working thus, alternately up the back.

This type of manipulation can be done over any localized area, particularly in the presence of nodules or localized tightness.

## Storms' Technique

Harold D. Storms of Toronto, Canada, developed a stroke that he used both for diagnostic and therapeutic measures, particularly for fibrositic nodules.

The cushions of the fingertips or the ball of the thumb do not slide under the skin; instead, they hold position on the skin, the short stroke being made possible by moving the connective tissue *under* the skin.

This stroke varies from the previously described friction strokes in that the direction of the stroke is always parallel to the muscle fibers, rather than circular or cross-fiber in direction. Storms specifies also that as soon as the spasm *begins* to soften, massage should stop for that day.

## Cyriax's Friction for Fibrositic Muscles

Cyriax recommends deep friction given to the site of the lesion, which may or may not be within the painful area outlined by the patient.

There are four ways in which one may use the hand to provide friction *across* the fibers of the structure being treated. Muscle, ligament, and joint capsule require friction administered perpendicularly to the long axis of the fibers composing them. The thicker and stronger the tissue, the greater the exactitude needed.

This can be done using the index finger crossed over the middle finger, the fingertips of the middle and ring fingers, opposed fingers and thumb in a pinching position, or superimposed thumbs, with the one thumb reinforcing the other.

## SUMMARY

Although there are many times when friction is not used at all in giving massage, there are other times when effleurage and petrissage merely prepare the tissues for the deeper application of friction. If one concentrates on working into this depth *gradually,* the patient will be able to tolerate more depth. By the same token, when the operator is "letting go," it should be gradual and so slow that the patient experiences no sudden change. The following discussion of tapotement will further develop the student's knowledge of massage technique. As previously stated, all techniques learned thus far should be interspersed when practicing tapotement since, until one has mastered the art of "bouncing off," the patient may take a slight "beating."

# ─12─

# Tapotement

Although tapotement is not used as often as the other massage techniques, it does have its place and requires practice to be able to perform it well.

Because of the indiscriminate use of tapotement in beauty salons and as often shown in motion pictures on prizefighters, and because of the unscientific claims that excess flesh can be "beaten off," many operators shun using it at all. However, it should not, because of this misuse, be ignored. If anything, emphasis on doing it correctly, and definition of its proper use, should be stressed.

Any series of brisk blows, following each other in a rapid, alternating fashion, come under the broad term of tapotement. Included under this heading are hacking, cupping, slapping, beating, tapping, and pincement.

## PURPOSE OF TAPOTEMENT

Tapotement is used when stimulation is desired. Because most massage is for purposes of relaxation, tapotement is often not a part of general massage routine. In athletics when stimulation is usually the purpose of massage, it plays a more important role. Occasionally, the apathetic patient may receive a slight stimulation and a pleasant sensation of well-being following massage that has been terminated with tapotement.

## APPLICATION OF TAPOTEMENT TO THE BACK

### Hacking

Before reading the following instructions, shake the hands, letting the wrist, hand, and fingers relax and "flip up and down." No attempt should be made to hold the fingers together or the hands or wrists in any particular position. If relaxation is complete, it will be noticed that the hands fall into a neutral plane of motion that neither supinates nor pronates the forearm (Fig. 12–1).

When relaxation is complete, an alternate direction of each arm can be started. One moves up as the other moves down, still keeping the hands relaxed and shaking them (Fig. 12–2).

Approach the patient, holding the hands so that the palms are parallel. Strike the back with a series of soft, but brisk blows, using the backs of the third, fourth, and fifth fingertips. Use both hands, alternating them and striking rapidly (Fig. 12–3). Done correctly, the effect is one of *pleasant* stinging and stimulation.

Progress from the hips upward to the shoulder and then back downward to the hips again. Tapotement should never be done over the kidneys.

## Cupping

This stroke is applied with the same rhythmical, rapidly alternating force, changing only the position of the hands to apply the blow with a cupped hand. Cup the hand so that thumb and fingers are slightly flexed, and the palmar surface contracted (Fig. 12–4). Strike the back with the palm of the hand. This presumably causes a slight vacuum with each blow and some people believe it may loosen the broad flat areas of scar tissue. If done correctly, it makes a rather loud noise that could be detrimental or useful, depending on the psychologic situation at hand.

## Slapping

In the same manner, but using an open rather than a cupped hand, strike gently but briskly with the fingers, rather than the palm of the hand (Fig. 12–5).

## Beating

The same stroke can be done using the hypothenar eminence of the hand, with the fist closed. Care should be taken to keep the force of the blows light and "bounding" in effect rather than jarring (Fig. 12–6).

## Pincement

Similarly, rapid, alternate, *gentle* pinching that picks up small portions of tissue between the thumb and first finger can be done (Fig. 12–7).

## Tapping

Tapping is done with the ends of the fingers, using sharp taps that make use of moderate fingernails, or padding the tap by using the pads of the fingers if the patient cannot tolerate the sharpness of the ends of the fingers.

## Quacking

This is done with palms together and fingers apart using the described tapotement technique.

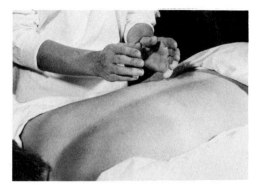

**Figure 12-1.** Starting position.

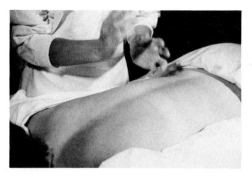

**Figure 12-2.** In motion.

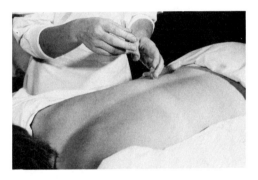

**Figure 12-3.** On contact.

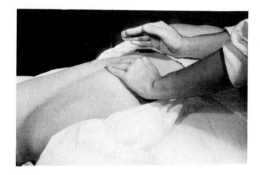

**Figure 12-4.** Cupping.

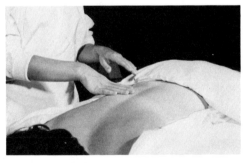

**Figure 12-5.** Slapping.

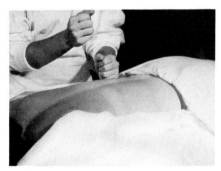

**Figure 12-6.** Beating.

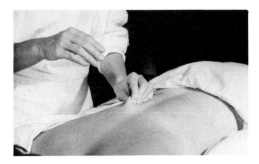

**Figure 12-7.** Pincement.

## Squishes

Cross the palms to form an air pocket, then "squish."

## Skritchies

Using thumb and forefingers, alternately pluck the surface of the scalp.

## SUMMARY

Any series of brisk blows following each other in a rapid alternating fashion come under the broad term of tapotement. They may be hacking, cupping, slapping, beating, tapping, or pincement. The purpose is usually to provide stimulation. These techniques need much practice to be applied with skill and if one cannot do them skillfully, the techniques should not be used at all.

# ──13──

# Vibration

Vibration was developed in Europe. Although it is described here for those who want to use it, it is this author's opinion that vibration can be given better with an electrical vibrator, with the exception of the very gentle vibration mentioned in treating peripheral neuritis and poliomyelitis.

A fine tremulous movement, made by the hand or fingers placed firmly against a part, will cause the part to vibrate.

## PURPOSE OF VIBRATION

Vibration is often used for a soothing effect, particularly in treating peripheral neuritis. The treatment follows the path of the nerve. Vibration for this purpose must be very gentle and rhythmical, using fine vibrations. It has been used in Europe for poliomyelitis patients with such delicacy that the vibrating hand does not even touch the part, but merely flutters above it.

## APPLICATION OF VIBRATION TO THE BACK

Use the same draping and position previously described. Place one hand anywhere on the back with the fingertips slightly apart. The rhythmical, trembling movement comes from the whole forearm, through the elbow, but the waist and finger joints are kept stiff. The elbows should be slightly flexed. This vibrating motion should be more up and down, than side to side. Heavy pressure should be avoided, especially if used with peripheral neuritis patients.

## VARIATIONS OF VIBRATION

When following the path of a nerve for a soothing effect, an effleurage type of stroke done with just the fingertips is employed, adding the vibration to the light effleurage stroke. Pressure can be so light that there is almost no contact of the hand with the part, and the vibrating hand moves almost without contact. With extremely hypersensitive cases, this technique has been credited with bringing a soothing effect.

### Shaking

Another variation of vibration in a much coarser degree is useful for patients who have difficulty relaxing. It often helps to pick up the muscle belly (especially the biceps or gastrocnemius) and gently shake it back and forth. It is also helpful at times to shake the entire limb gently in order to encourage relaxation.

## SUMMARY

Vibration should not be used at all if one has not put the time and effort into learning to do it well. Done well, it can be extremely soothing, but done poorly it will only cause frustration and impatience on the part of both patient and operator. It is difficult to learn well, and seldom used in America. Emphasis given to this technique must be decided by the operator.

This concludes the basic strokes of massage. The following chapters describe how these techniques can be applied to any part of the body for a variety of therapeutic effects.

# — 14 —

# Application to Parts of the Body

As previously emphasized, each patient will display different symptoms even though the diagnosis for different patients may be the same. The following suggestions pertaining to each of the different areas of the body point out some general approaches that make it easier for the operator to apply massage. Trained, sensitive fingers searching for muscle spasms, nodules, and painful areas should be able to locate the unique symptoms of each patient.

## MASSAGE OF THE BACK

Using the positions and draping described in Chapter 9, effleurage and petrissage should be given to the following muscles or muscle groups:

- Erector spinae
- Latissimus dorsi
- Gluteals
- Trapezius
- Rhomboids
- Levator scapuli

Light effleurage to all the above will make the operator aware of tense or painful areas to be given more detailed consideration later in the treatment. All strokes should follow the muscle fibers. Any or all of the techniques learned previously can be applied. A variety of strokes and patterns can be selected to treat the individual complications that each patient may have.

## MASSAGE OF THE LOW BACK

### Position

When positioning the patient for low-back involvement, the operator should consider putting the spine in slight flexion by placing a pillow under the abdomen with the patient face-lying. Some patients cannot lie comfortably in this position. If moving is difficult or impossible, the operator must adapt the technique so that the patient can be treated side-lying or even lying flat on the back. Therefore, effleurage and petrissage should be practiced with the patient lying in all positions. This involves applying the strokes at different angles. Consequently, the operator may need to adjust the working height by stepping on or off a low platform.

When lying on one side, the patient should have the top leg well supported. The top arm should be supported in a position where the operator is sure the patient is not using it to help maintain the side-lying position. Pillows under the leg and arm will not only give them support, but also will keep the patient from falling forward when pressure is applied to the back.

### Draping

Draping is no different in principle for any of these positions. A sheet or towel should keep any part that is not being treated covered and warm.

### Application of Technique

Because of heavy fascia in the low back area, many patients can tolerate rather heavy pressure. The piriformis is often in spasm and only deep friction through relaxed gluteals can exert any pressure on it. The amount of direct mechanical pressure that can be applied on this muscle is debatable.

## MASSAGE OF THE GLUTEI

Many people will be sensitive to massage of the glutei, therefore some special approaches should be discussed.

### Draping

As little of the area should be exposed as possible. Only that which is necessary should be left uncovered. The operator can often work under the sheet. If only one side is involved, a sheet can be placed so it covers the entire other half of the body, including the gluteal cleft.

### Application of Technique

The operator can help the patient adjust to the touch of his or her hands by working on either the lower extremity or the back, stroking gradually toward the gluteal area. This is contrary to the usual approach of massaging the proximal area first. The purpose of reversing this procedure is to help the patient adjust to treatment of this area.

Strokes to this area need to be heavy due to the large muscle mass. They should follow the direction of the muscle fibers for each of the gluteal muscles. Follow the usual sequence of effleurage, petrissage, and friction where indicated. Deep effleurage strokes that go around the acetabulum and the tuberosity of the ischium should be included. It is difficult to reach through this large muscle mass to palpate the piriformis, which is often in spasm, but with relaxation of the gluteals it can sometimes be accomplished.

Friction can often be tolerated about the lumbosacral and sacroiliac regions but should be done carefully because these areas are often sensitive. Friction should also be done over the area of the greater sciatic notch, the ischial tuberosities, and the area between the iliac crest and the greater trochanter.

If the patient must lie on his or her back, the problem for the operator is to reverse the technique for applying pressure downward to that of reaching under the patient and applying pressure upward. Effleurage is fairly easy to do in this fashion, but petrissage is much more difficult. One hand can effect the circular motion of the usual two-hand petrissage, progressing up the back. Friction is also easy to apply, using the tips of the fingers with the palm facing the patient, working with the typical small circles of friction or with a cross-fiber technique.

Practice of massage to the back should be done with the patient in all positions, even seated with the head resting on a pillow against the treatment table, because patients with back involvement often find lying down very difficult.

## MASSAGE OF THE CERVICAL AND THORACIC SPINE

### Position

Patients requiring massage of the thoracic or cervical spine are often more comfortable lying face down, with a pillow under the chest, and with the head supported by a small, rolled towel in a neutral position. Patients have a difficult time getting comfortable if they have pain in this area. One often discovers that the patient is better at finding a comfortable position than being told in which position to lie. If it is impossible to find a comfortable position lying down, the massage can be given with the patient in a sitting position, leaning on a pillow placed on the treatment table. Either position is acceptable. Possibly the sitting position is a little more convenient for the operator. The arms may be placed wherever they are comfortable as long as they do not support the weight of the patient and are relaxed. In some instances the head may be held supported with a Sayre head sling for support or slight stretching combined with massage. Some patients will be more comfortable in a back-lying position with the operator standing at the head of the treatment table.

## Draping

There should be no clothing on the upper back. Women may be given a hospital gown that opens down the back but protects the rest of the body if treated in a sitting position. If the patient is lying down, the draping is the same as it has been for the other techniques applied to the back.

## Application of Technique

All of the variations of effleurage described can be applied to this area. The three-count stroking of the upper trapezius (*see* Fig. 9–4) is especially useful. Stretching can be applied to the upper trapezius. Use one hand to stabilize the head and the other to give a deep effleurage stroke that goes from the origin to the insertion of the upper trapezius. Pressure should be deep enough to stretch the muscle fibers but never deep enough to cause pain. Care should be taken that the stabilizing hand does not push the head away. It maintains good alignment of the cervical spine, serving to hold the head still so that the stretch is accomplished by pushing the shoulder downward, not by pushing the head away.

## Sayre Head Sling and Stretching

In cases when the Sayre head sling has been prescribed, effleurage strokes for the upper trapezius can be applied while the patient is receiving traction from the head sling.

Care should be taken to ensure that pressure is so placed that normal alignment of the cervical spine is not displaced.

Verbal instructions for relaxation will assist the patient in getting maximal benefit from this type of treatment (*see* Chapter 6).

All petrissage techniques can be adapted to this situation, even the one-hand petrissage, which can be used on the upper trapezius. Two-hand petrissage can also be done on the muscle mass of the upper trapezius, which can be grasped with the hands molding over the anterior aspects of the muscle. If deep petrissage is done with upward progression toward the head, it should be followed by deep effleurage strokes downward to assure good venous return. Watch the complexion of the patient; if the face is flushed, only downward pressure should be used.

Friction may be used as previously described (*see* Chapter 11), following up the spine on either side of the spinous processes all the way up to the occiput. Any involvement of the upper back or neck is apt to cause marked tenderness at the occipital protuberance. Friction, therefore, is cautiously applied around the tendinous insertion, or not done at all if the patient cannot tolerate this type of pressure.

Mennell refers to "sensitive deposits" that can be felt under the exploring hand of the operator.[1] These deposits are often found in the muscle bel-

---

[1]James B. Mennell. (1945). *Physical treatment by movement, manipulation and massage* (5th ed.). Philadelphia: Blakiston's Son, p. 474.

lies in this area and can be treated as described by Mennell or Storms. Storms' methods have already been discussed (*see* Chapter 11). Mennell advocates the use of frictions that begin gently at the periphery of the sensitive area and gradually approach the center of it. This should be followed by deep petrissage. Cross-fiber manipulation may also be used in a similar fashion.

Although tapotement and vibration may be used, these strokes are not routinely part of the treatment.

## MASSAGE OF THE CHEST

### Position
The patient should be back-lying with due consideration for the relaxation of all muscles that originate or insert from the chest. Slight flexion at the knees would tend to relax the abdominals. Pillows under the arms will relax the pectorals. A pillow under the head should relax the muscles of the neck.

### Draping
A towel or sheet should cover the side not being treated to keep the patient warm and comfortable.

### Application of Technique
Other than tapotement, any or all of the techniques described may be applied to the chest. Because of the many types of surgery or injuries that could be treated in this area, no particular approach to special muscle groups can be outlined. Involved muscles should be treated by groups. Scar tissue and limited shoulder movement, especially following mastectomy, may often be the major concern. Stretching should be applied if the shoulder has been held in protective splinting, which leads to tightness. In this event, consideration should be given to those posterior muscles that may also be tight.

## MASSAGE OF THE ABDOMEN

### Position
The patient should be back-lying with the knees in slight flexion and supported so that the hip flexors and abdominal muscles are relaxed. The head may be resting on a pillow.

### Draping
A towel or sheet should cover the upper part of the patient, and another one the lower part of the patient so that only the abdomen is exposed.

## Application of Technique

Orders are almost never received for abdominal massage. There was a time when it was ordered for constipation. This author does not recommend it, but includes it for those who might want instruction.

Gentle effleurage strokes should be used to accustom the patient to the touch of the operator. All strokes should follow the direction of the colon, as it ascends on the right, crosses, and then descends on the left. Gradually increase pressure (but never too heavily). Light petrissage may follow the same pattern followed again by effleurage.

It is usually easier for the operator to stand on the patient's right side.

Friction, with precaution against going too deeply, can then follow. Use circular strokes that follow the direction of the colon. Complete the treatment with light effleurage in the same direction.

**Caution:** Abdominal massage could cause serious complications in the event of pregnancy, appendicitis, or other abdominal disorders.


## MASSAGE OF THE UPPER EXTREMITY

### Position

Range of motion in the shoulder joint may be the deciding factor as to whether the patient will be treated in a sitting or lying position. If there is tightness of the pectorals, but not inhibiting pain, it is well to treat the patient sitting with the arm supported. This puts a slight stretch on tight muscles while the patient is being treated. The amount of stretch can be increased by raising the height of the arm or lowering it if it cannot be tolerated. If severe pain, as with bursitis, prevents this position, the arm may rest on a pillow in the patient's lap or on a lower table. Some patients are more comfortable lying down.

If the hand or wrist is involved, the hand is usually supported by a small roll or towel so that it rests with the wrist slightly extended. If relaxed, the fingers will rest in partial flexion. This position also puts the fingers slightly off the table, which protects the fingertips from bumping on the table if they are hypersensitive.

### Draping

Only the arm being treated should be left uncovered. A towel or a sheet may be used to cover the patient in such fashion that it will not slip, particularly if the patient is in a sitting position. If the entire arm is to be treated, the draping should cross the shoulder not being treated and be fastened securely with a safety pin. Sleeves of the patient should never be pushed up. The shirt or blouse should be taken off to prevent tight clothing from inhibiting the venous return.

### Application of Technique

The greatest change noticed in adapting the strokes to the arm and hand is in the position of the operator's hand. As previously described, the hand is open to cover the wide surfaces in the back. On the arm and hand a closer position will be used to encompass the smaller area with close contact, using either the C or the V position.

## Upper Arm

Muscles or muscle groups to be considered in massage of the upper arm would include those of the cervical and upper back if the shoulder is involved. (See pages 95–97 for general procedures.) These muscles are often tense from muscle splinting to avoid pain in the injured or involved arm. If so, they should also be treated. Muscles of the arm include the pectorals, serratus, deltoid, triceps, and biceps. In addition to massage for each muscle or muscle group, the joints should be considered. Care should be taken not to place deep pressure into the joint or over bony prominences.

## Elbow and Forearm

The patient is seated. The arm rests on a pillow, providing flexion of the elbow and pronation of the forearm. Give two short strokes toward the insertion of the biceps, first the medial side then the lateral side. Stroke from distal to proximal along the medial border of the upper third of the brachioradialis. Stabilize the elbow joint from the back. Follow the upper third of the ulnar side of the palmaris longus stroking toward the origin. Stop before the epicondyle. Give long strokes that pull from the distal two thirds of the brachioradialis. Change hands.

Give long strokes on the ulnar side of the palmaris longus, beginning at the lower third of the arm and stopping at the epicondyle. Change hands.

Stabilize the wrist. Pull over the ulnar border of the flexor carpi ulnaris. Stop before the condyle. Stroke on the dorsal side of the arm along the edge of the extensor digitorum communis from the lower third of the origin. Bimanual "widening" of the elbow joint is done with the patient's elbow flexed. Hold the olecranon and pronator teres in one hand, and the brachioradialis in the other hand. Pull outward with both hands (Figs. 14–1 and 14–2).

## Lower Arm

In the lower arm, the flexors of the wrist and fingers can be treated as a group. The extensors comprise the other major muscle group to be treated. Those muscles crossing both the elbow and the wrist should be considered. Both of these joints should be included in the massage and any limited range of motion should be *gently* stretched using effleurage strokes that encourage increased range of motion.

If some of the muscles of the upper arm, such as the biceps, are involved due to muscle splinting or casting positions, the massage should include treatment of them also.

## Application of Technique

To perform massage strokes, the operator uses the soft pads of the fingers to pull over the full length of the muscles with some depth from distal to proximal.

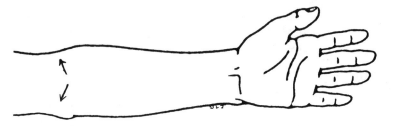

**Figure 14-1.** Stretching technique of the elbow.

As illustrated in Figure 14–2, the first stroke pulls over the lower third of the flexor carpi radialis. The second stroke pulls over the palmaris longus. The third stroke pulls over the flexor carpi ulnaris (Fig. 14–3).

## Hand

A common problem of an inexperienced operator is the *overstretching* of the capsule in the small joints of the fingers. The fingers need to be stretched *gently*. A gentle, steady pull, combined with slow effleurage wherein the operator's first finger surrounds most of the finger, while the thumb covers the dorsal aspect, will feel good and also be beneficial to the patient. However, the "popping" of the joints can be very harmful and should be avoided. A Mennell type of passive motion that gently encourages active motion and increases the range of motion can be combined with massage of the fingers. *Little good can come from overstretching.* It tears the tissues and causes increased swelling and pain.

The fingers are so small that massage is difficult. It must be practiced until it can be done well. Hand injuries are common and the swelling and limited motion that accompanies such injuries need treatment.

All strokes previously described can be adapted to these smaller areas and must be mastered. Elisabeth Dicke's strokes so completely cover all aspects of massage to the hand that they are included under Bindegewebsmassage (*see* Chapter 24). For general massage, the author prefers that all strokes proceed from distal to proximal, whereas Dicke describes strokes from proximal to distal.

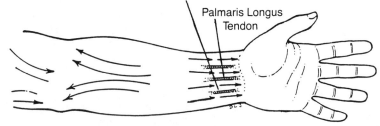

Tendon of Flexor Carpi Radialis

Palmaris Longus Tendon

**Figure 14-2.** Application of massage to the elbow and forearm.

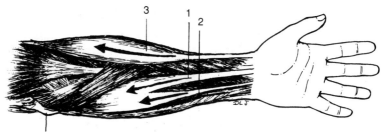

**Figure 14-3.** Stroking the palmaris longus, flexor carpi radialis, and flexor carpi ulnaris.

Medial Condyle

## MASSAGE OF THE LOWER EXTREMITY

### Position

The person receiving massage to the lower extremity should be lying down with the leg in a neutral position or elevated in the event of swelling. There should be support at the knee and at the ankle. The foot should never be allowed to drop into plantar flexion, even though it is not necessarily involved. A pillow or drop-foot board should support the foot at about 90 degrees of dorsiflexion.

The person may be face-lying if most of the treatment pertains to the posterior aspect of the leg. In this case the feet should be off the end of the treatment table and the lower leg supported so that the knee is in slight flexion, unless stretching of the hamstrings or gastrocnemii is indicated.

### Draping

With an injured lower extremity, it is often difficult for the patient to get out of pajamas or trousers. This can easily be handled by asking the patient to loosen the top of her or his pajamas or trousers. Then advise her or him to hang onto the top of the sheet. Standing at the foot of the bed, reach under the sheet and pull the trousers off. Always check to be sure the patient has a tight hold on the sheet or both the sheet and trousers will come when the trousers are pulled.

Occasionally, there is demand for what is jokingly called "diaper" draping (Fig. 14–4). This can be tactfully managed by handing the patient a towel and asking him or her to place it so that it goes between the legs, covering the patient, both front and back. The patient can do this while protected by the sheet, working under it, or the operator can leave the room while the patient does the draping.

### Application of Technique

Mold the hands to the contours of the leg in applying effleurage and petrissage to the muscle groups involved. Care should be taken not to carry any strokes too high on the medial thigh. All of the principles mentioned in massage of the upper extremity also apply to the lower extremity.

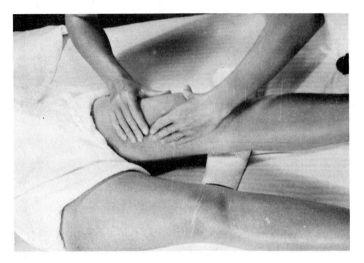

**Figure 14-4.** "Diaper" draping. Massage to the upper leg.

## Upper Leg

Muscle groups that should be considered in massage of the upper leg include the gluteals if the hip is involved. The hamstrings, adductors, abductors, and quadriceps should be treated as groups and are usually involved in injuries to the hip or knee, or fractures of the thigh. The hip flexors are seldom massaged, but in the event of hip-flexion contractures they would benefit from treatment.

Gentle stretching of the hamstrings and gastrocnemius may be done. Using both hands just above the popliteal space, lightly hold the tendons of the hamstrings with the fingertips. Lift and supinate both hands, gently stretching the tendons (Fig. 14–5). This same technique can also be used for the two heads of the gastrocnemius, just below the popliteal space, but never working deep into the popliteal area.

In cases of injuries to the leg, the patella often lacks normal mobility. In cases of arthritis, care should be exercised so as not to work too deeply with friction around the patella. Use one hand to stabilize the patient's leg,

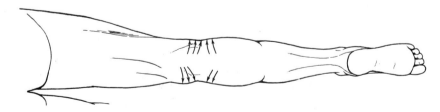

**Figure 14-5.** Application of massage to the upper leg.

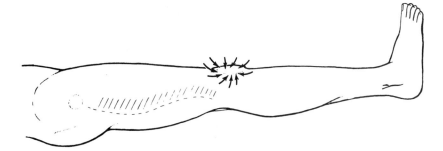

**Figure 14-6.** Friction-like strokes to the patella.

while using the other hand to perform short, deep friction-like strokes that follow the border of the patella (Fig. 14–6).

Pivot-like strokes, in which the heel of the hand acts as a pivot and the fingers stroke around the borders of the patella, can also be used (Fig. 14–7).

## Lower Leg

In the lower leg, the tibialis anterior, tibialis posticus, the peroneals, and the gastrocnemius comprise most of the muscle masses that are to be treated as muscle groups. These muscle groups can be effleuraged and petrissaged in preparation for detailed attention to be given to any particular problems.

Use bimanual stroking of the Achilles tendon, working from distal to proximal, from the medial and lateral malleolli upward over the gastrocnemius. The hands flex the foot slightly as they stroke (Fig. 14–8).

Stroke the peroneus longus and brevis, around the malleolus, and proximally up the leg. Stabilize the leg with one hand (*see* Fig. 14–9a).

In the same fashion, stroke the tibialis posticus and around the malleo-

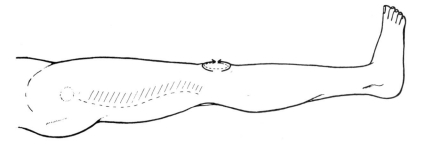

**Figure 14-7.** Pivot-like strokes to the patella.

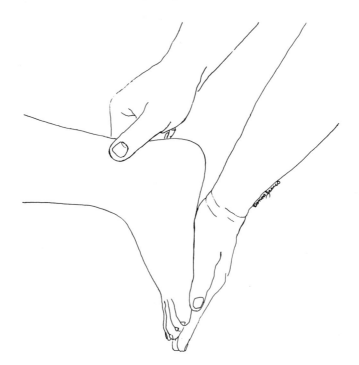

**Figure 14-8.** Stroking to the Achilles tendon. One hand massages the foot while the other hand flexes the foot.

lus (Fig. 14–9a). Complete the series by stroking bimanually both of these areas at the same time.

## Foot

All the principles brought out in the discussion of massage to the hand, particularly the special care taken when working with small joints, apply to massage of the foot. Stabilize the foot with one hand.

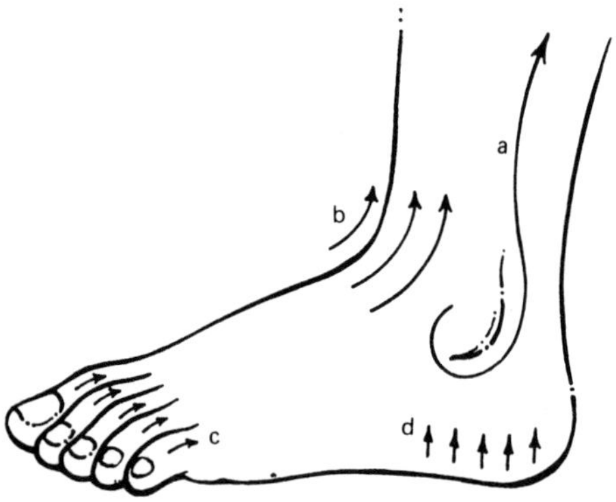

**Figure 14-9.** Massage to the lower leg and the foot.

Use little strokes moving distal to proximal across the front of the ankle joint. Dorsiflex the ankle while stroking (Fig. 14–9b).

Apply short small strokes between the metatarsophalangeal joints, going from distal to proximal, then medial to lateral (Fig. 14–9c).

If the toes are involved they will be massaged exactly as the fingers.

Deep short strokes should be made just in front of the heel, from the arch along the side of the foot, starting laterally and working medially. The same should be done going the other way, starting medially (Fig. 14–9d).

Short strokes can be made across the bottom of the heel. Deep stroking of the plantar fascia can be done with long strokes that cover the longitudinal arch from the heel up to the metatarsophalangeal joint, using the knuckles to achieve deep pressure (Fig. 14–10). Foot reflexology will be discussed in Chapter 25.

Plantar stroking may also go across the muscle fibers at right angles to the longitudinal arch (Fig. 14–10b).

Bilaterally stretch both the top and bottom of the foot with a rolling motion of the hands; up and out on the proximal part of the foot. On the distal part of the foot, reverse direction to stretch the forefoot (metatarsal arch) in the opposite direction (Fig. 14–11).

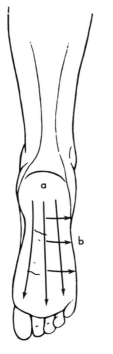

**Figure 14-10.** Plantar stroking across muscle fibers.

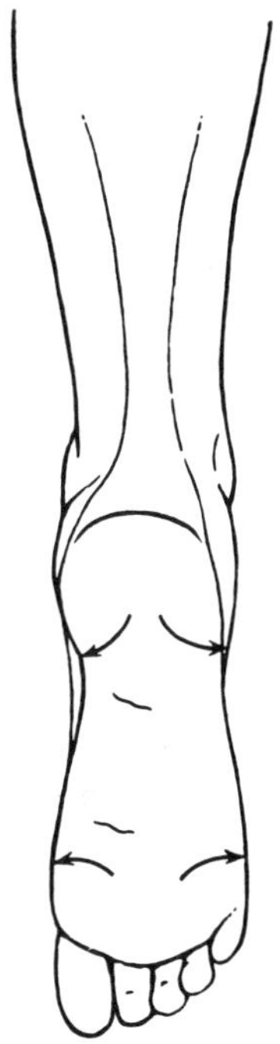

**Figure 14-11.** Bimanual stretching of the foot.

## MASSAGE OF THE FACE

### Position

The patient may be lying down or seated, as preferred. The operator stands behind the patient.

### Draping

A small towel or head band may be used to keep the hair away from the face during the treatment.

### Application of Technique

In cases of Bell's Palsy, the involved side of the face is often stretched, being pulled by the well muscles on the opposite side, especially around the mouth. In giving treatment, both sides should be massaged, as the side of the face *not* paralyzed will also have muscles that are tight. Support to lessen this pull should be given with the hand not being used to massage, alternating as both sides are treated.

Bimanually stroke across the forehead, from the hairline down to just above the eyebrows, moving from the center of the forehead toward the temple (Fig. 14–12a).

Stroke gently using the pads of the fingers from the lateral side of the eye into the hairline of the temple (Fig. 14–12b). Follow the upper eyebrow, stroking from medial to lateral toward the temple (Fig. 14–12c).

Repeat the same, following the lower rim of the eyebrow (Fig. 14–12d). Repeat the stroke just below the eye (Fig. 14–12e).

Apply short strokes upward between the eyes (Fig. 14–13a). Pull from the involved side to the uninvolved side over the bridge of the nose. Reverse the direction (Fig. 14–13b).

Bimanually stretch the nose, stroking from the center to each side. Work all the way down to the very tip of the nose (Fig. 14–13c). Bimanually stroke the zygomaticus, working from just under the eyes toward the mandible, stroking from front to back (Fig. 14–14). Soft strokes directly over the closed eyes of the person, pulling from the nose slightly over to the temple, can be very relaxing.

Petrissage can be performed with two fingers in the smaller areas and with the thumb opposing the fingers over the fleshier parts of the face.

*Gentle* friction directly over the temples is especially good for a headache. Friction all around the hairline will ease tension caused by frowning or muscle tightness that originates there. With finger and thumb, the bridge of the nose can be stretched by pulling it outward.

For all these strokes, gentleness must be emphasized, and care taken not to put pressure directly over the eyes. Contact lenses should be removed.

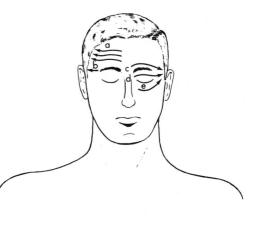

**Figure 14-12.** Massage to the face.

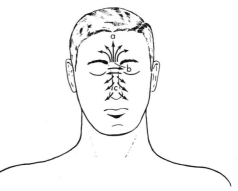

**Figure 14-13.** Massage between the eyes.

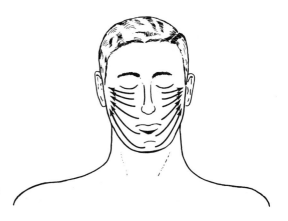

**Figure 14-14.** Stroking the zygomaticus.

## SUMMARY

Each person will develop his or her own combinations of strokes for all parts of the body. This chapter provides many suggestions to assist the student in developing skill in adjusting the hand, whether the area is large or small. The hand can more easily be studied in Chapter 24, in which Dicke's method is discussed. The author, however, prefers strokes to proceed from distal to proximal instead of from proximal to distal as in Dicke's procedure.

# PART III

# Use of Massage for Various Healing Purposes

# 15

# Use of Massage in Nursing

The development of Therapeutic Touch is central to nursing because the nurse with trained and sensitive hands can greatly enhance the quality of patient care. In controlled studies Dolores Krieger has demonstrated the positive physiologic effects of touch[1] (*see* Chapter 5). Furthermore, through the "laying-on of hands" one can communicate the uniquely human *concern* of one individual for another in an act that incorporates an intent to help or heal the person so touched. Since 1976, Dolores Krieger has published *The Therapeutic Touch*. She has become well known for her study and development of the technique, and she continues to teach her healing methods throughout America in workshops, on radio, television, and in many published articles. People interested in this field of massage should attend her workshops and study her text in detail.[2]

Massage provides a valuable approach that can comfort the distraught patient if the nurse applying the treatment extends concern both verbally and tactilely. The patient will feel the interest and compassion extended for his or her welfare.

With skillful hands, nurses will gain the confidence of their patients. Discomfort is relieved and positive attitudes are developed. Physiologic, mechanical, and reflex effects are accomplished. Such a massage need not take more than five minutes. In fact, more than five minutes may do more harm than good.

Patients confined to bed develop areas of physical discomfort due to

---

[1]Dolores Krieger. (1976, April). Nursing research for a new age. *Nursing Times*, 1.
[2]Dolores Krieger. (1979). *The therapeutic touch.* Englewood Cliffs, NJ: Prentice-Hall.

inactivity. Chapter 4, Part I, explains the physiologic reasons for this discomfort and tells how massage can relieve this type of distress.

Any or all the techniques described in this book may be used. Massage
of normal tissues that are not involved with the patient's pathologic condition can often relax the patient who is restless from long hours in bed.
Nurses who can skillfully execute basic massage techniques will earn the
gratitude of their patients.

## MASSAGE OF THE BACK

If the patient has been back-lying for quite a while, massage to the back is
recommended. In preparing the patient for rest and sleep, the entire massage should be done in a slow, rhythmical, relaxed fashion. This contact
presents an excellent opportunity to build confidence in the patient and promote feelings of security and well-being. Although empathy can be shown
without words, a soothing voice combined with light rhythmical stroking
can also strongly motivate the patient toward restful sleep.

Muscular tightness through the shoulder and neck muscles due to uncomfortable resting positions and increased tension in the patient can be
relieved with petrissage to this area. Strokes should work from deep to
light. Strokes that go downward from the head toward the coccyx are more
restful than those that go upward. The relaxing stroke described in Chapter
10 will often leave the patient almost asleep.

## MASSAGE FOR PRESSURE AREAS

Patients who lie quietly in bed due to paralysis or weakness should receive
a good massage to areas where pressure is apt to cause decubitus ulcers.
Combined with frequent changes of position and proper resting positions,
massage can help prevent the formation of decubitus ulcers.

Deep strokes that bring blood to the area should be applied each time
the patient is moved. Here again, this need not take a great deal of time, but
the results are most gratifying.

Common sites for decubitus ulcers are found over the sacrum, the back
of the heels, elbows, and knees. When the patient is turned, one can readily
see where pressure has recently been placed because the area will turn red.
Effleurage and petrissage may be applied with depth. Stroking *toward* the
pressure areas will encourage capillary dilation. Friction can also be applied around the pressure area. Once a decubitus ulcer has developed to an
acute phase, massage alone will be of little use and should not be attempted
by the nurse.

## MASSAGE FOR THE IMMOBILIZED PATIENT

Patients who have been immobilized by traction or casts often become uncomfortable because of positions that must be maintained. The patient with a leg in traction may complain of discomfort to the back or neck.

With precaution against moving the injured limb, massage to the uncomfortable area can relieve much of this discomfort.

## SUMMARY

Except for the many nurses who have studied Dolores Krieger's methods of Therapeutic Touch, the professional nurse in a hospital setting does very little real massage. The routine back rub now seems to be missing from standard care. When one considers the stress level of most patients who are hospitalized (and stress reduction is the objective of massage), one feels a certain sadness that this brief but relaxing touch no longer seems necessary for routine care. Any nurse, any time, who can find time to console even one patient through massage, however brief, should be encouraged to do so.

Research indicates the importance of extending *truly caring attitudes* from one human being to another. Massage given by a caring person can enhance the quality of patient care because physiologic, psychologic, and reflex effects can be accomplished by the laying-on of hands. Attitudes of compassion can be expressed through massage, even if only for five minutes of a nurse's time.

# 16

## Massage as Used by Physical Therapists

During World War II, physical therapy was primarily a "hands-on" treatment that depended more on heat, massage, and exercise for the ill or injured person. Many army-centered schools developed and trained physical education majors to become therapists. During and after the war many of these therapists worked with infantile paralysis patients before the Salk vaccine was perfected and, indeed, a good share of that regimen included heat (hot packs), massage, and exercise for weakened muscles.

The bizarre muscle weakness pattern from infantile paralysis led to a great need for exact knowledge of kinesiology.

Shortly thereafter, the greater need for developmental progress of muscle function led therapists to study neurophysiologic approaches to normal functions. With infantile paralysis now controlled, there was a greater need for therapists to concentrate on the developmental approaches for birth-damaged infants and children who have many problems throughout their entire life. Many of the techniques for dealing with infantile paralysis were also found to be helpful for brain-damaged people. Neuromuscular facilitation techniques requires a firm understanding of neurophysiology.

The emphasis of the role of the physical therapist shifted toward treating the patient in an entirely different way. Massage became of less and less importance to their treatment.

Historically, as this change took place, the ever-present need for people to be touched in a caring way became a demand, to the point that schools of massage therapy began to develop. Today it is known that the effects of massage on the patient are so beneficial that the most progressive physical therapists now rely on this ancient method of treatment.

At present, many departments of physical therapy in medical centers hire massage therapists to offer treatment for those patients for whom massage is a definite indication for treatment. Some physical therapists who feel the need for hands-on therapy will attend schools of massage therapy on a postgraduate level.

The author published the first massage text of this type in 1960 when physical therapists truly felt that the sharing of touch, "hands on body," was more than just a physical therapy modality. Through massage one could penetrate to the depths of one's very being.

On a spiritual level, the benefits of massage are difficult to define. It touches the *life force*—that essence that the whole is greater than the sum of its parts. Knowing that somebody cares can mean the difference in wanting to live when the going gets tough.

Massage and touch is essential for all ages. Unfortunately, when it is needed the most in later life it is often given less. In today's aging society, the touch that comforted people as babies and children begins to diminish in adulthood. Single adults living alone are found more frequently in our society. Even massage cannot replace the active life style after people retire, but it helps.

Arthritic joints can safely be treated with gentle massage and stretching if inflammation is not present. Special attention should be given to the comfortable position of the one being treated due to inflexibility. Attempts should be made to maintain the full range of motion in all joints. Caution should be used if there are contraindications (such as cardiovascular problems).

## SUMMARY

No amount of scientific research has to this day been able to prove the importance of the unconditional loving touch. There will always be scientific minds demanding proof.

It is sincerely hoped that this trend will reverse itself. In a sense, this book has a mission: to remind people that massage therapy, which was used extensively since before humans could write, can be one of the most important tools anyone involved with health care, and especially physical therapy, can utilize.

# —17———————————

# Massage for Animals

Concern for the well-being of animals almost always leads to stroking, scratching, and otherwise demonstrating affection. Therefore, one might as well know a few things about how to do it properly. This chapter will discuss ways to massage animals to accomplish more than random caresses and ensure improved physiologic health at the same time.

As explained earlier (*see* Chapter 4), correct massage will increase hemoglobin, assist the venous flow of blood, encourage lymphatic flow, reduce certain types of edema, and provide gentle stretching of tissue to prevent decreased range of motion and increase metabolic balance in muscles by ridding them of toxic products caused by underactivity or overactivity.

The same indications and contraindications for massage apply whether working with animals or people, because basically they have similar (albeit different) anatomic and physiologic structures. For the same reason, all the basic principles of massage apply (*see* Chapter 3), as well as the basic techniques of effleurage, petrissage, friction, tapotement, and vibration (*see* Chapters 9 through 13).

## MASSAGE AND ACUPUNCTURE FOR HORSES

Acupuncture works especially well with animals for their chi points are very comparable to those of humans.

Jack Meagher, a physical therapist, became interested in deep massage for horses. He wrote about the fact that, regardless of the size and shape of the package, muscle and joint problems are the same. They range from 10-lb show dogs to 1500-lb horses; from 120-lb marathon runners to 280-lb NFL linebackers. The same problems occur in every sport for the same reasons. The physics and physiology of motion and the cause of strain-type injuries are always the same. It is the location of these spasms at the end of the muscle that is the reason deep massage not only brings blood to the area but also releases histamine and acetylcholine into the tissue resulting in hyperemia that will last long enough to benefit the tissue through follow-up exercise.

Cross-fiber manipulation can be applied by holding this pressure and moving back and forth in a sideways movement across the grain of the muscle. This type of friction spreads and separates the fibers in preparation for their normal motion of shortening and lengthening. Pressure is always applied directly inward toward the bone. The hand and fingers should move as one. If the hand slides over skin, the value of depth will be dissipated.

Identifying stress points is easy. Normal tissue gives under the hand and there is no pain. Sharon Gale of Coventry, Conn, studied with Meagher and became very skillful in locating stress points and bringing relief from pain to many horses. The horse recognizes immediately that this treatment "feels good" and is going to help.[1]

In Figure 17–1 Gale is stretching a foreleg after having relieved the stress points involved with the particular problem. One can easily see that the horse is indeed content and cooperative. Gale claims horses have gone to sleep while being massaged. They also extend their stride when running, to the point at which one horse actually knocked off his front shoe with an overextended forward reach with his hind leg.

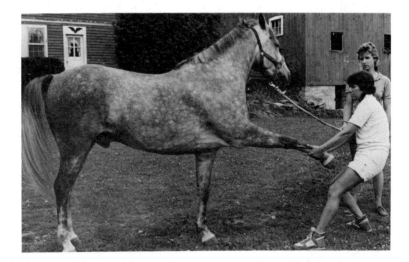

**Figure 17–1.** Massaging animals such as horses can improve their physical performance as well as relax them. (*Photo by Fran Funk.*)

---

[1]Personal consultation with Sharon Gale, March, 1987.

To apply massage techniques to animals it would be helpful to have at least a basic knowledge of the particular structure of the bone and musculature of each particular animal being given a therapeutic massage. To adapt any of the methods discussed in this text is not beyond the imagination. The pet will feel similar reactions as those of humans to include relief of pain, relaxation, and mood elevation.

## INTERACT WITH THE ANIMAL

Animals pick up feelings and attitudes. Communication, especially with animals, is mostly nonverbal—using such cues as tone of voice, facial expression, posture, and other behavior. Because animals do not use speech, body signs are even more important as communication and can include smell as well.

Consideration should also be given to direct mind-to-mind communication. Although this theory lacks objectively tested proof, which the medical profession desires before giving its approval, it is considered a valid phenomenon by many sensitive people.

The author once had a dog named Punch, who would do exactly as instructed when Punch lived in Storrs, Conn, and the author was living temporarily in New York City. After reading *Kinship with All Life*,[2] she was inspired to try ESP with Punch, although Punch was "visiting" a home the author had never seen.

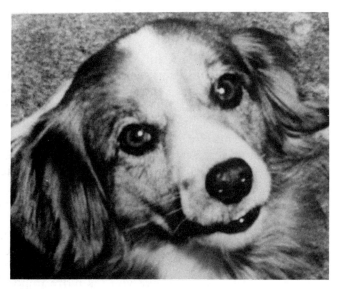

**Figure 17-2.** Punch.

[2]J. Allen Boone. (1954). *Kinship with all life*. New York: Harper & Row.

While driving toward Connecticut, Tappan first tried to visualize exactly where Punch was and what the dog was doing. The image she received consisted of Punch asleep on a small rug. So she first sent the all-encompassing message of unconditional warm love by concentrating on this emotion for about 15 seconds. This was followed by a cheerful instruction of "Wake up, Punch! Wake up!" for another 15 seconds. When she "felt" she had Punch's attention, Tappan sent this message to the dog, "Go to the window. Go to the window and look outside. I'm coming, Punch. I'm coming to pick up my little dog. Here I come." When she could visualize that Punch was responding, she added, "Now go to the front door and bark. Bark! Bark! Let them know you want to go *out!*" Again, she concentrated on this message until she felt the message had been received, then she sent, "Now sit on the curb and wait for me. I'm coming, Punch . . . Love . . . Here I come . . . Love . . . I'm almost there . . . "

Such mental activity was continued until Tappan drove up to the house to find Punch waiting at the curb for her.

Upon entering the house, she found Mr and Mrs Everett wide-eyed with excitement saying, "Do you know that dog knew you were coming?" The author feigned innocence, saying, "Well, what makes you think so?" and they replied, "Punch was asleep on that little rug over there. Suddenly she sat up, looked about, ran to the window, and looked outside, then ran to the door, barking to be let outside. Then she sat on the curb and waited until you came!" "My my," said the author, "Punch must have ESP!"

From that time on, for the rest of Punch's life she responded promptly to any and all instructions from her mistress whether she was 2 miles or 100 miles away. This was confirmed by several other people who cared for Punch at various times while the author traveled away from home. Punch—upon receiving ESP instructions from Tappan—would awaken her caretakers at five o'clock in the morning by barking at the door insistently, until she was let out, and she continued to bark until the neighbors complained. Punch could even selectively wake up different people she lived with at 5 AM until each of those people called Tappan long distance and asked her to "Cut that out!" These people included absolute "disbelievers" until each was aggravated into submission of belief!

Therefore, although many people are skeptical of ESP in any form, and scientists are busy trying to prove it does or does not exist, this author strongly believes that the power of thoughts and feelings can bridge the communication gap between animals and people. Owners of animals should visualize the white healing light of love to their pets, combined with touching and stroking of any kind.

The owners of pets may also *cause* many problems. If the owner is nervous, unloving, or sick, the animal will pick up on the negative feelings and become ill or emotionally upset itself.

To think "I love you" is more important than the vocal saying of the words, especially if it is sincerely felt by the person sending the message.

Directing thoughts toward healing has been known for centuries. Research has proven in double blind studies that 92.8% of those animals treated by love and light improved, whereas improvement was seen in only 73.7% treated by the usual medical methods.

So, massage animals—anything from gerbils to horses. Be calm and relaxed and positive in their presence and while treating them. Let go of worry and fretting about the pet's problems and trust in the healing power of nature. Provide necessary veterinary care. While at home, create a safe, peaceful, quiet, comfortable space, physiologically and psychologically.

Talk to your pets every day, normally, as if your words are expected to be completely understood. Encourage and expect health for your pets and mentally visualize them as being well and healthy, playing happily and purring contentedly. Imagine every cell as radiating and healthy. Be positive and encouraging, being careful not to support any illness by fawning and fussing over them when they show symptoms.

Give pets a reason to *live* by providing love and appreciation. Demonstrate that the pet contributes to the household; be sure the animal feels wanted.

# ——18————————————

# Sports Massage

A careful search of the literature reveals the fact that all the usually applied techniques of sports massage are the same as those already discussed in the previous chapters. There are, however, particular aspects to consider when working with the athlete.

Physical therapist Jack Meagher, coauthor with Pat Boughton of *Sports Massage*,[1] was a pioneer in the field of sports massage, as well as the massage of animals (*see* Chapter 17). Sports massage differs from other types of massage in that the treatment should be done preferably before an injury occurs. It considers anything less than maximum efficiency to be a problem and the lead-in to more serious problems. Sports massage goes beyond the problem itself to the underlying cause.

One looks for a bit of knotted tissue that restricts motion because of the pain it causes. In all cases, the exact causative spot must be located. The tissue involvement is symptomatic. Heat of any kind cannot reach nor affect a deep causative lesion (spasm), nor will contractive currents release a part being held in full contraction.

Although rest is essential for a period of time following an actual injury, rest becomes counterproductive by allowing the spasm to achieve permanent status when adhesions form.

A spasm requires three things to ensure its release:

1. A hyperemia (circulatory increase) to soften the tissue.
2. Therapeutic motion to the spastic fibers to restore normal motion.
3. Proper follow-up exercise.

---

[1] Jack Meagher and Pat Boughton. (1980). *Sports massage.* New York: Dolphin/Doubleday.

Most spasms can be found at the ends of the muscle, which can be released with deep massage therapy. Direct pressure applied to the exact spot (stress point) in spasm with the thumb or finger tips will provide the necessary hyperemia. Blood is then drawn to the exact spot. Histamine and acetylcholene are necessary. A spasm is rigid and it is painful when deep pressure is applied. One must depend on the reaction of the person being treated. Muscle spasms are real, they are there, and they can be felt.

By the time stress points can be identified by palpation of tense tissue, a spasm of the muscle has begun to form. Common sense will alert the therapist to eliminate spasms before they cause major problems.

As with all specialties, sports massage should be studied under an experienced specialist before one claims to be able to conduct sports massage. At the same time, any graduate of a good course in massage should have all the fundamental skills described in this text.

The well-rounded training program of any sport should include massage. The coach should know how to make use of massage for conditioning before activity, and how to prevent or reduce lameness following extreme activity. This does not mean that all athletes should be given a conditioning massage before every game.

There are apt to be instances when massage might help some outstanding member of the track or swimming team break a record. In such cases, massage might add extra nourishment to the vital muscle groups to make this effort worth the coach's time.

## PRECONDITIONING FOR MAXIMUM ACTIVITY

Meagher's text discusses the importance of massage for athletes of all kinds, from tennis players to runners. He claims that you can gain 20% in performance, that it is a mistake to ignore even slight injuries, and urges people not to suffer silently. Better yet, he advises people to keep themselves in good condition through massage, exercise, acupuncture, and homeopathy. Through his efforts, massage has become indispensable for everyone from weekend amateurs to Olympic champions by contributing that extra boost to help speed recovery, lower stress, promote greater endurance and flexibility, prevent injuries, and enhance body awareness.[2] This concept is far from new. It has been used since the days of the ancient Roman gladiators.

Treatment should be given the day before the expected activity. The athlete should plan on a half hour of complete rest following this treatment and an evening that ensures minimal exertion and a good night's sleep.

Massage should be preceded by a brisk needle shower, from warm (about 110°F; 45°C) to cool (80°F; 25°C).

---

[2]Information extracted from Mirka Knaster. (1986, July). *The wholistic athlete,* Brooklyn, MA: East–West, p. 44.

With the person lying prone, give a brief general massage that covers the back. Work from light effleurage rather quickly into deep effleurage and petrissage of all the large muscle groups of the back. Encourage relaxation and make sure that the resting position is comfortable.

When sufficient general relaxation has been obtained, massage can be begun on the muscle groups that will be used most in the activity planned for the coming day. Thus, if the event requires running, the legs would be carefully massaged with deep effleurage of the gluteals, hamstrings, and gastrocnemii, working to deep kneading of all these muscle groups, not forgetting the anterior aspects of the leg, particularly the quadriceps and anterior tibial group.

When each muscle group has been carefully massaged, the whole extremity should be gone over again with long sweeping effleurage strokes that follow from the heel all the way up the back of the leg and over the gluteals.

Brisk tapotement of any type leaves the patient with a feeling of tingling well-being.

In the same manner, if the coming event involves the arms, the latter part of the massage should consider mostly the thoracic spine and arms. If the activity involves the use of all four extremities, the total body should be considered, doing first one side and then the other.

Those who have had experience have come to realize the value of putting essential muscle groups into a good metabolic state previous to extremes of activity. There is less tendency toward lameness following the activity.

The purpose of preconditioning is to ready the muscles for exertion. The purpose of massage following such activity is to carry away the waste products that have collected due to this exertion. It does not require stimulation, for the muscle has been stimulated and is now tired, and seeks rest and inactivity. If the muscle is exhausted enough, it will not perform its normal activity of "milking" these by-products into the venous return. The person who has put forth a supreme effort is physically tired, and at this stage exercise cannot accomplish the desired exchange in metabolism because the muscles themselves are too weary to profit by further exercise.

Therefore, the purpose at this point is to "wring out" the muscle and mechanically do this job of milking for it. Gently kneading the muscle free of such by-products will allow it to take advantage of the fresh supply of blood and lymph which automatically follows the massage.

Since stimulation is not desired, a warm shower should precede the massage. The rate of the stroke is much slower. (Remember the flow of lymph is slow and sluggish.) Watch the more superficial veins and give them time to refill following the effleurage stroke. If muscle soreness is involved, pressure must be regulated so that it is firm enough to squeeze out the muscle without provoking a muscle splinting type of protective tensing.

Tapotement is not indicated unless the individual requests it, for now the aim is not one of stimulation or preparation, but rather, rest and complete relaxation. This in itself allows a normal return of new and nourishing blood to the tired muscle and minimizes the tightness and spasm that come from stiff and sore muscles.

If any tightness or spasm is present, and there is not injury to the muscle, such as rupture or hematoma, active normal range of motion may be attempted. If there has been any sign of injury to the muscle, no treatment of any kind should be attempted without consultation with a physician.

## CHARLEY HORSE (MUSCLE CRAMP OR SPASM)

If a muscle is asked to do more than it has been conditioned to do, and extreme activity is undertaken without proper warm-up exercises or a building-up to be able to do a task of sudden activity, the result will be sudden, painful spasm of the muscle. The muscle is not able to meet the chemical exchanges to keep its metabolic balance.

The name *charley horse* has also been given to the painful spasm that results from severe kicks or blows that are accidentally received in competitive activity.

Upon occasion, the muscle will actually rupture and hematoma can readily be seen. If there is any indication that these spasms or cramps have been severe enough to cause bleeding within the muscle belly or tearing of the tendon, no measures should be taken to massage or exercise the part until advised to do so by a physician.

If, however, there is cramping due to inability of the muscle to meet the metabolic needs and stresses placed upon it, effleurage and petrissage can assist the muscle back to normalcy. If the muscles do go into spasm, it is an indication that these muscles are not in condition for activity. Conditioning exercises will avoid repetition of such "casualties."

General knowledge of all the massage techiques will be valuable information for those in the field of sports. Precautions should be taken to avoid massaging any injury that should not be treated by these techniques. The major uses of massage in athletes presented in this chapter will lessen chances of injury, prevent unnecessary lameness, and prepare muscles for peak performance.

The importance of the physiologic effects (discussed in Chapter 4) becomes realistically important as sports massage aims toward maintaining homeostasis for all athletic endeavors.

## SUMMARY

Massage has become an integral and important necessity in the field of sports medicine. All the massage techniques discussed in this text may be used with particular attention related to indications and contraindications. It is imperative for any athlete to incorporate massage as an integral part of the training regimen.

# — 19

# Massage of Infants and Children

Because the skin absorbs nutrition, vegetable or olive oil is especially useful for baby massage. The mother holds the baby on her lap with as much skin to skin contact as possible between herself and her baby. The room should be warm (for example, a bathroom following a bath), as should the mother's hands. Follow an effleurage sequence working outward from the center to cover the entire body of the baby. Rhythm, love, and gentle caring are an important part of this daily routine.

## MASSAGE OF PREMATURE INFANTS

Ruth Diane Rice, a nurse, psychologist, and specialist in early child development, received her Ph.D. degree from the University of Texas at Austin, after completing a research study in sensorimotor stimulation of premature infants. Rice developed a specific stroking and massage technique that she used in an experimental study of 30 premature babies. The mothers were taught this technique, which includes touching, movement, and the sound of a heartbeat, similar to the conditions the baby experienced in the womb.[1]

Such infant research has shown that touching, movement, and sound stimulate the nerve pathways and cause the following to occur:

1. An increase in myelination, dendritic processes, and Nissl substance in the brain cells resulting in a speeding up of neurologic growth.

---

[1]Ruth D. Rice. (1975, November). Premature infants respond to sensory stimulation. *American Psychiatric Association Monitor, 6,* 8.

**127**

2. A higher output of the growth hormone somotrophin, causing faster weight gain.
3. An increase in the output of the hypothalamus, which serves as a general arousal center, leading to increased cellular activity and endocrine functioning.

The development of Rice's stroking and massaging technique and the success she has had using it have brought her national and international recognition from persons in medicine, nursing, psychology, and child development.

Rice believes there must be revolutionary changes made in the care of newborn infants and in parent–child interaction if the high incidence of emotional disturbance, learning disabilities, hyperactivity, and many other disorders that have their origins in infancy are to be prevented.

Research shows that massaging premature infants can help them catch up developmentally with full-term infants. Massaged babies gained 47% more weight than others who were not massaged; they were more active, more alert, and performed better overall.

"Walking fingers" or "creepie-crawlies," in which the parent's fingers crawl spider-like up the back usually make the baby laugh.[2]

## THE IMPORTANCE OF TOUCH

Leboyer speaks eloquently about the importance of an infant's first touch.

> A word about the hands holding the (newborn) child.
> It is through our hands that we speak to the child, that we communicate.
> Touching is the primary language.
> "Understanding" comes long after "feeling."
> Among blind people, this touching has never lost its subtlety and importance.
> Immediately, we sense how important such contact is, just how important is the way we hold a child.
> It is a language of skin-to-skin—the skin from which emerges all our sensory organs. And these organs in turn are like window-openings in the wall of the skin that both contains us and holds us separate from the world.
> The newborn baby's skin has an intelligence, a sensitivity that we can only begin to imagine.
> It is through this skin that the unborn child once knew its entire world: that is, its mother. It was through the entire surface of its back that it knew her uterus: our backs are, literally, our past.
> Now the baby is born. And suddenly this contact is gone. Forever.
> Hands touch him. Hands so unlike the uterus in temperature, in weight, in the way they move, in their power, and in their rhythm.

---

[2]Robert J. Trotter. (1987, January). The play's the thing. *Psychology Today, 21,* 27.

This is the baby's first contact with the unknown, and with the new world, with that which is "other."

And our hands that touch and hold the baby, these unknowing, unfeeling hands, have no understanding at all of everything the baby has experienced until this moment.

Our hands are instruments of our intelligence, our will.

They are obedient to the muscles. Voluntary, agile muscles. Their movements are quick, brief, almost brusque.

And terrifying to the infant who has experienced only the slow internal rhythms of the womb.

How could the child *not* panic at this new kind of touch? And how, then, ought we to touch—to handle—a newborn baby?

Very simply: by remembering what this infant has just left behind. By never forgetting that everything new and unknown might terrify and that everything recognizable and familiar is reassurance.

To calm the infant in this strange, incomprehensible world into which it has just emerged, it is necessary—and enough—that the hands holding him should speak in the language of the womb.

What does this mean?

That the hands must "remember" the slowness, the continuous movement of the uterine contraction, the "peristaltic wave" the child grew to know so well during the final months before its birth.

This is another reason why it is necessary to first place the child flat on its stomach—so that, in massaging it, we "speak" to its back.

And what should our hands say? Exactly what the mother and her womb have been saying.

Not the womb as it was during final labor, not the violent womb that expels and banishes. But the womb of the early, happy days.

The womb that pressed slowly, tenderly. The womb that embraced. The womb that was pure love ... What is needed is neither a brisk rubbing motion nor a caress, but a deep and slow massage.

Our hands travel over the infant's back, one after the other, following each other like waves. One hand is still in contact as the other begins. Each maintaining its steady rhythm until its entire journey is concluded.[3]

*Infant Massage,* by Vimala Schneider[4] combines Swedish massage and the massage she learned while studying in India in 1973. By 1976, when her own baby was born, she had studied Swedish massage and began to combine these two systems as she massaged her own child. Thus motivated, she became the author of this excellent text, which is recommended for all people professing to be complete massage therapists.

Bonnie Prudence[5] discusses deep finger pressure using the thumb to locate painful trigger points in babies. Since babies cannot talk, people need to be ingenious to discover why they cry. After checking all the usual causes for a baby's cry without success or relief, the idea that pain could be the

[3]Frederick Leboyer. (1976). *Birth without violence.* New York: Knopf, pp. 59–62.
[4]Vimala Schneider. (1982). *Infant massage.* New York: Bantam.
[4]Bonnie Prudence. (1984). *Pain erasure.* New York: M. Evans, p. 150.

cause occurs; it follows that palpation would be a good way to find the problem.

She relates a case in which the baby did not walk or stand. The concerned parent consulted doctors who, after careful examination, could find no real problem and suggested bracing. Tender trigger points were found in the gluteals, adductors, and hamstrings. The mother was instructed on the precise treatment: apply deep pressure at each point for about 5 seconds. In 2 weeks the baby was walking.

Not all cases are this extreme. A search for tender spots could also indicate acupuncture points that are tender (*see* Chapter 20). People with knowledge of acupuncture could readily relieve a baby's headache, tummyache, and in many cases, minor problems by the use of finger pressure to the acupuncture point.

## SUMMARY

Massage of infants is an imperative part of parenting that can be done by both the father and the mother—or even older brothers and sisters. Touching stimulates the infant's understanding of being loved and cared for, and strengthens the baby's need to be comforted.

# PART IV

# Variations of Massage Techniques

# 20

# Finger Pressure
# to Acupuncture Points

**HISTORY OF ACUPUNCTURE**

Although the origin of Chinese medicine is lost in antiquity, it is assumed to have developed from folk medicine. It has many aspects in common with other Oriental traditions, such as Indian herbal medicine and Persian medicine. The origin of acupuncture is, however, unique to the Chinese branch of Oriental medicine.

The earliest known text on acupuncture is the *Nei Ching*, or *Classic of Internal Medicine*, traditionally ascribed to the legendary Yellow Emperor (Huang Ti, believed to have lived from 2697–2596 BC). The *Nei Ching* remains the basic reference on the subject and is the foundation for all development in acupuncture to the present century.

The ancient Chinese became aware of an increased sensitivity of certain skin areas (called points) when a body organ or function was impaired. It was observed that in all patients the same skin areas became hypersensitive in the presence of a specific illness or organ dysfunction. Consequently, some of the relationships between various internal organs and their functions were observed and established. These were defined and explained in terms of a complex philosophical hypothesis that attempted to relate all the observed phenomena.

Acupuncture has a known history antedating Christianity by 2000 years. Over the course of centuries a long line of ancient practitioners belonging to a people noted for meticulous visual observation were able to establish the existence of a number of meridians and their relationships with various physiologic functions. Fundamental to the concept of meridians in Chinese medicine is not only their function as imaginary lines linking a series of points on the skin that become sensitive in the presence of organic or functional disorders, but also their function as actual "energy pathways." The Chinese word for energy is *chi* (often spelled *ki*).

This energy is considered to circulate throughout the body in a well-defined cycle, moving in a prescribed sequence from meridian to meridian and from organ to organ, flowing partly at the periphery and partly in the interior of the body. Like the Western concept of "nerve-energy potential" or the *prana* (life force) of Indian philosophy and medicine, *chi* is a dynamic force in constant flux.

Acupuncture was introduced to the West in the seventeenth century by Jesuit missionaries sent to Peking. Since that time, several attempts have been made to promulgate this therapy of the Orient, with varying degrees of success. Not until the French sinologist and diplomat Soulié de Morant published his voluminous writings on acupuncture in the 1940s did Western physicians have a sound basis for study and application of this ancient system of healing.

Under the impetus of de Morant's work, acupuncture associations and study groups were established in many Western countries, among them France, Italy, Britain, West Germany, Argentina, and the Eastern European nations. Many countries now actively support research programs in the physiology and application of acupuncture, notably the USSR, the People's Republic of China, North and South Korea, and Japan.

Acupuncture is of growing interest in the West, but it is also undergoing a resurgence of serious study in the Far East. In China, acupuncture is an integral part of the nation's medical practice.

The field of acupuncture treatment is that of impaired body functions, as opposed to actual lesions. In the case of a patient with diabetes, for example, if there is no actual tissue degeneration in the islets of Langerhans, acupuncture can be extremely effective. Even if lesions have formed and are well established, the pain, discomfort, and other symptoms caused by them are greatly relieved by acupuncture. It is impossible, however, to obtain complete and lasting relief of a functional problem that has an organic substratum by use of acupuncture.

One of the primary functions of acupuncture is to directly affect the energy level, and therefore the functioning, of the internal organs by either stimulating or depressing their actions.

## MERIDIANS—A MYSTERY?

Oriental philosophy and medical science believe that meridians are a system of pathways, or channels. The meridian system provides for a continuous flow of vital energy and nutrients to all parts of the body. Although there seem to be neither definite anatomical meridian structures throughout the body, nor a specific relationship to existing systems as we know them, Robert Tsay observes that the "... meridian system may differ somewhat from the nervous system, the blood circulation and the endocrine system, but it is also possible that it is intimately related to these three systems."[1] The theory of the meridians is the basis for diagnosis and treatment. According to Tsay, ". . . it is impossible for the physician to differentiate symptoms, or to prescribe accurately the exact treatment for a patient without using this theory as a guide or basis. This is the reason it is necessary for the student of Chinese medicine to first study the theory of the meridian system. It is as important as the student of Western medicine having to first learn anatomy, physiology, and pathology."[2]

The 12 regular meridians are listed in the order of vital energy and nutrient flow, with rare exception, as follows:

1. Lung (L)
2. Large Intestine (LI)
3. Stomach (St)
4. Spleen (Sp)
5. Heart (H)
6. Small Intestine (SI)
7. Urinary Bladder (UB)
8. Kidney (K)
9. Pericardium (P)
10. Triple Warmer (TW)
11. Gall Bladder (GB)
12. Liver (Liv)

Governing Vessel (GV), and Conception Vessel (CV), the first two extra meridians, are the thirteenth and fourteenth of the most used meridians.

GV covers the total posterior midline of the body and a midline portion of the head anteriorly. CV covers the remaining anterior midline portions of the head and body.

As listed, circulation of energy and nutrients starts through L, continuing through each of the meridians in succession. From Liv the energy flows to and through the L meridian again. The complete cycle takes twenty-four hours and repeats continually throughout life. Branches of the meridians allow for the vital energy transport from one meridian to the other.

## Features of the Meridians

No real anatomical vessels can be found by dissection. Two components of circulation go through the meridian circulatory system: *Chi*, the invisible circulation of the vital energy, and *Hseuh*, the visible circulation, including blood and lymph.[3]

Meridians are named according to (1) the organ that is controlled by the

---

[1]Robert C. Tsay. (1974). *Textbook of Chinese acupuncture medicine, General introduction to acupuncture*, (Vol. 1). Wappinger Falls, NY and Las Vegas: Assoc. of Chinese Medicine and East-West Medical Center, p. 44.
[2]Tsay (1974), p. 52.
[3]Tsay (1974), p. 40.

energy flow, i.e., lungs, stomach, spleen; (2) the function of the energy, i.e., GV, Regulating Channel (RC), and Motility Channel (MC); and (3) Yin or Yang.

In a Yin meridian, energy mainly flows upward. In a Yang meridian, energy mainly flows downward. The Oriental Yin and Yang theories compare in some ways to what Western scientists call positive and negative elements, which exist in every atom. Even when atoms are split, particles still maintain positive and negative charges. Only very recently have scientists thought that anything at all could exist without a positive and a negative particle.

The Oriental philosophy believes that the solar system is a large universe with its Yin and Yang. All lives are part of it, and the human body is like a smaller universe within this particular galaxy. Since an atom contains its Yin and Yang, a cell therefore contains its Yin and Yang, and an organ contains its Yin and Yang. Any individual body that may be deemed a unit must also contain its Yin and Yang.

Upon review of the literature on meridians, one will find that various authors name the system differently. For example, meridians may be called channels or pathways. The meridians may also be named in other ways, e.g., lung (L) is also pulmonary (PU); large intestine (LI) is also colon (C); stomach (St) is also gastric (GA).

There are the following types and numbers of meridians: (1) twelve regular meridians; (2) eight extra ones; (3) twelve chief branches and twelve muscle branches; (4) fifteen liaison vessels; and (5) twelve cutaneous liaison vessels. The 14 meridians most often used are the 12 regular ones and the two extra meridians, GV and CV.

As vital energy and nutrients flow during the 24-hour cycles, there are two-hour intervals when a maximum of vital energy is reached in each of the 12 regular meridians. Intervals start with 0300–0500 in the meridian. This maximum vital energy time is considered the best time to treat pathologies of that meridian. As McGarey points out,

> If asthma attacks occur, particularly at night, it is felt best to treat the problem during that two-hour period between three o'clock and five o'clock A.M. In the Western world, it does not seem likely that this would get done outside an emergency room very often, but nevertheless, this is the rule of acupuncture and should be recognized as such for whatever value it may have at some future time in one's experience.[4]

Flow in the meridians follows three specific cycles within the 24-hour period. Each cycle contains four meridians, as grouped within the 12 meridians. Figures 20–1 through 20–8 illustrate the four meridians in each cycle, with the direction of the flow indicated. Figures are shown with upper ex-

---

[4]William A. McGarey. (1974). *Acupuncture and body energies.* Phoenix: Gabriel Press, p. 35.

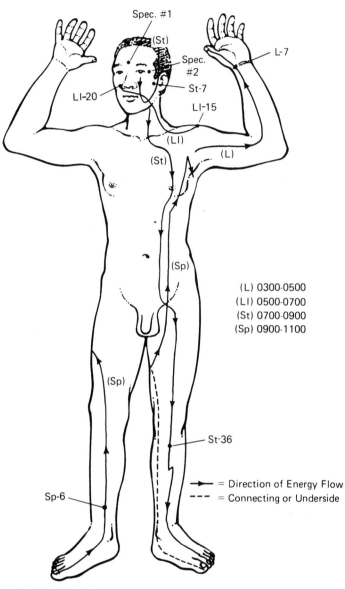

**Figure 20-1.** First cycle anterior.

tremities raised above shoulder height to better illustrate the *up* and *down* direction of the vital energy and nutrient circulation. In each figure the right side is used as the right side in both anterior and posterior views. Remember, the meridians are bilateral, therefore, the circulation is duplicated on the left.

A total of 20 enlarged dots are located on the meridians in all but one of the figures (Fig. 20–3). These indicate acupuncture points, each named

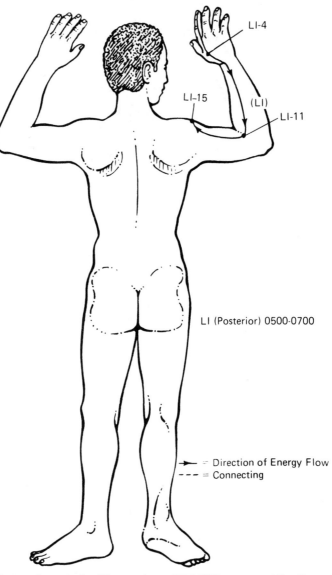

**Figure 20-2.** First cycle posterior. The numbers, 0500-0700, represent the time of day.

according to the meridian on which it is located. The 20 points have been selected by specialists in the field. They are thought to be most effective when used, in various combinations, for treating common painful areas, i.e., head, shoulder, low back, and leg. Selection was made from the 642 points found on (1) the 14 most used meridians—361; (2) special acupuncture points, also called extra points—171; and (3) new acupuncture points—110.[5]

---

[5]Huang Min Der. (1975). Medical seminar at Chinese acupuncture science research foundation, Taipei, Taiwan, R.O.C.

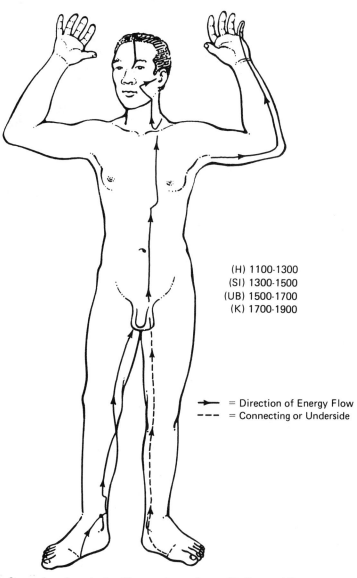

(H) 1100-1300
(SI) 1300-1500
(UB) 1500-1700
(K) 1700-1900

→ = Direction of Energy Flow
--- = Connecting or Underside

**Figure 20-3.** Second cycle anterior. The numbers given with the meridians represent the time of day.

Each of the three cycles illustrated has the following features: each cycle is composed of four different meridians; each meridian is either a hand or a foot meridian; each is either a Yin or a Yang meridian; and each has a two-hour interval when a maximum of vital energy is reached, called the maximum energy time. Each cycle also has a definite sequential direction of vital energy and nutrient flow through the four meridians of that cycle. Flow starts through a Yin meridian, going *up* from the chest area to the *hand*; then from the hand, *down* toward the chest and head area via a

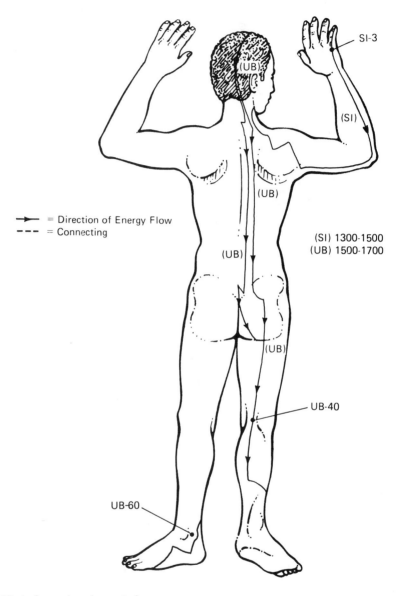

**Figure 20-4.** Second cycle posterior.

Yang meridian; from the head area *down* a Yang meridian to the *foot*; and then from the foot, *up* to the chest area via a Yin meridian. Then flow continues to the next cycle Yin meridian in the chest. Features of the three cycles are included in Table 20–1.

Governing vessel and CV, the thirteenth and fourteenth of the most used meridians, are illustrated in Figures 20–7 and 20–8. The former also shows the combined posterior acupuncture points, whereas Figure 20–8, CV,

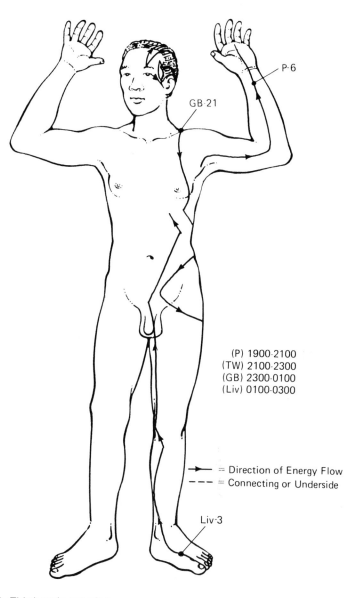

**Figure 20-5.** Third cycle anterior.

shows the combined anterior acupuncture points. For example, GV 26, one of the 20 most used acupuncture points, is seen on Figure 20–8.

Meridians are connected, in couples, through 15 points, called Lo Meridian Points. Liaison vessels serve as links between coupled meridians. As Tsay describes them, "Coupled meridians, composed of a Yin meridian and a Yang meridian, are closely interrelated as an inseparable body. Three couples are on the hand, and three on the foot. Couples may evidence identical

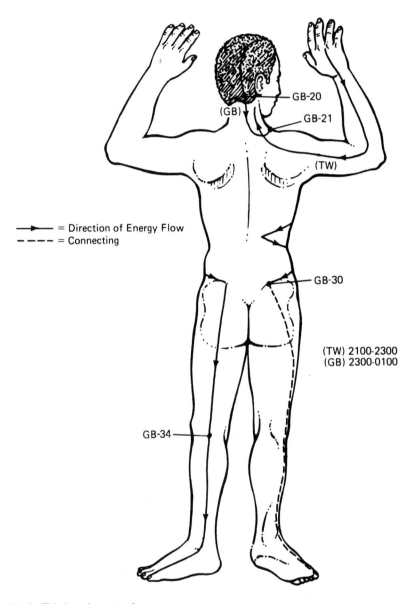

GB-20

(GB)

GB-21

(TW)

⟶ = Direction of Energy Flow
- - - - = Connecting

GB-30

(TW) 2100-2300
(GB) 2300-0100

GB-34

**Figure 20-6.** Third cycle posterior.

symptoms, and can be treated at the same meridian points."[6] (Meridian and acupuncture points refer to the same points.)

The meridian system is built anatomically in a nonspecific system functioning to balance all aspects of the human body: mental, digestive, reproductive, nerve, and circulatory processes; internal and external organs; and

[6]Tsay (1974), pp. 78–79.

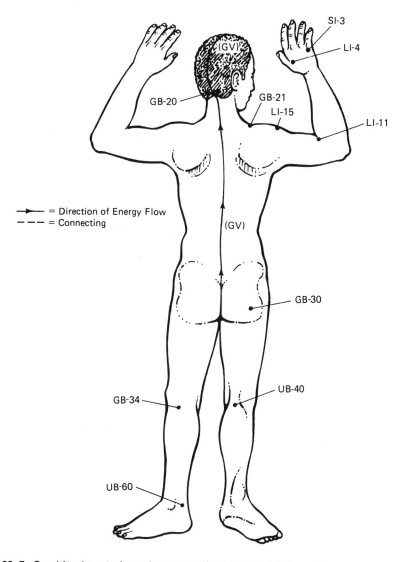

**Figure 20-7.** Combined posterior points; posterior portion of GV meridian.

energy, nutrition, and consciousness. Tsay notes, "Viewing meridians as lines—it is possible to see that many meridian pathways run closely parallel to the pathway of one or more main nerve branches. The anatomical relationship of the bi-meridian points with blood vessels are (sic) also very close, but not as close as with the nerves."[7] In order, then, to understand the workings of the body, to recognize symptoms of dysfunction, and to prescribe treatment, persons studying Chinese healing arts need the same basic

[7]Tsay (1974), p. 61.

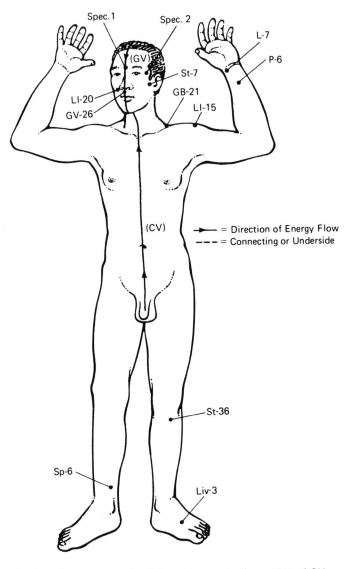

**Figure 20-8.** Combined anterior points; CV meridian; anterior portion of GV.

knowledge of the meridian system as those persons studying Western healing arts need anatomy, physiology, and pathology.

## PHYSIOLOGY OF ACUPUNCTURE

Studies proving that the electrical excitability of nerves can be reduced *solely* by acupuncture needles have been done on animals and humans (*see* Chapter 6 for a discussion of David Mayer's work).

**TABLE 20-1. THE THREE DAILY CYCLES OF THE MERIDIANS**

| Meridian (abbr.) | Hand or Foot | Yin or Yang | Maximum Energy Time[a] | Flow: Up or Down | Points Located on Figures |
|---|---|---|---|---|---|
| **First Cycle:** | | | | | |
| (L) | Hand | Yin | 0300–0500 | Up | (L) 7 |
| (LI) | Hand | Yang | 0500–0700 | Down | (LI) 4, 11, 15, 20 |
| (St) | Foot | Yang | 0700–0900 | Down | (St) 7, 36 |
| (Sp) | Foot | Yin | 0900–1100 | Up | (Sp) 6 |
| | | | | | Special points #1, #2[b] |
| **Second Cycle:** | | | | | |
| (H) | Hand | Yin | 1100–1300 | Up | |
| (SI) | Hand | Yang | 1300–1500 | Down | (SI) 3 |
| (UB) | Foot | Yang | 1500–1700 | Down | (UB) 40, 60[c] |
| (K) | Foot | Yin | 1700–1900 | Up | |
| **Third Cycle:** | | | | | |
| (P) | Hand | Yin | 1900–2100 | Up | (P) 6 |
| (TW) | Hand | Yang | 2100–2300 | Down | |
| (GB) | Foot | Yang | 2300–0100 | Down | (GB) 20, 21, 30, 34 |
| (Liv) | Foot | Yin | 0100–0300 | Up | (Liv) 3[d] |

[a]Energy time is the time of day when the available energy is at a maximum.
[b]Points located on the anterior are shown in Figure 20-1, and on the posterior in Figure 20-2.
[c]Points located on the anterior are shown in Figure 20-3, and on the posterior in Figure 20-4.
[d]Points located on the anterior are shown in Fgiure 20-5, and on the posterior in Figure 20-6.

In 1975, Frederick Kerr, Department of Neurologic Surgery at Mayo Clinic in Rochester, Minn, reported a study he conducted using rats.[8] The first rat was given acupuncture to Ho-Ku, Large Intestine 4. This reduced its trigeminal nerve excitability by 75%. The second rat was given no acupuncture, but was given a blood transfusion from the first rat with an acupuncture needle in his Ho-Ku. The result was that the second rat showed considerable lowering of excitability in its trigeminal nerve.

It has been shown that acupuncture points can be located with electrical apparatus, and that electrical resistance of the skin is consistently lower at acupuncture points. Acupuncture point areas often are tender, small nodules. Moreover, temperature differences in acupuncture points have been demonstrated with infrared photography.[9]

Needling sites also seem to correspond with the "Head Zones" discovered by Sir Henry Head in the 1800s. Pain resulting from pathology of the viscera is often referred to clearly definable areas on the body surface known as "Head Zones." These zones closely relate to the twelve acupuncture meridians and are associated with the same organs.[10]

Organs receive their autonomic nerve supply primarily from the homolateral part of the nervous system. Connective tissue changes can therefore be found on the corresponding part of the body surface. The liver, gall blad-

[8]Frederick W. L. Kerr. (1975, September 29). Conference at the University of Connecticut Health Center.
[9]McGarey (1974), p. 11.
[10]M. E. Armstrong. (1972, September). Acupuncture. *American Journal of Nursing*, 1582.

der, duodenum, ileum, appendix, ascending colon, and hepatic flexure receive their nerve supply mainly from the right. The heart, stomach, pancreas, spleen, jejunum, transverse and descending colon, sigmoid colon, and rectum receive their nerve supply mainly from the left.

Changes relating to the bladder, the uterus, and the head can be found in the middle of the back. Changes relating to the lungs, bronchi, kidneys, suprarenal glands, and ovaries can be found on the corresponding side of the back. Conditions affecting the nerves or vessels of either side of the body will cause changes on the corresponding side of the back.

The changes that can be observed visually may be grouped under what have for many years been called "trigger points." These include drawn-in bands of tissue, flattened drawn-in areas of tissue, elevated areas giving the impression of localized swelling, atrophy of muscles, hypertrophy of muscles and bony deformities, especially of the spinal column. Many trigger points seem to correlate with acupuncture energy points. According to this theory, pathology in muscles results in tenderness in the muscle, as well as its associated tissues and organs.

It has been evidenced that if the anatomical meridian is cut, the stimulation of an acupuncture point is not transmitted to other points of the same meridian beyond the level of the cut, and the internal organ with which the meridian is associated is not influenced by treatment with acupuncture.[11]

The word acupuncture combines two Latin words, one being *acus* meaning needle. Therefore, those who use the term acupressure for finger pressure on the acupuncture energy points are in fact saying "needle pressure," which is not at all what they intend to imply. The other word is *punctura*, which means pricking. Therefore, the term acupuncture means needle pricking or the insertion of needles into specific points of the body known as acupuncture points. The following discussion considers how these points can also be effective in massage by applying finger pressure.

## TECHNIQUE OF APPLYING FINGER PRESSURE TO ACUPUNCTURE POINTS

When using finger pressure on acupuncture points, more than just the amount of pressure applied should be considered. As with all massage, the degree of pressure must be judged in relation to the tolerance of the patient. For this particular technique the more pressure the patient can tolerate, the greater the effectiveness of the treatment. However, judgment must be exercised when dealing with acute pain, swelling, local injuries to the area being treated, and systemic complications. Deeper pressure will probably be needed if the complications are chronic.

---

[11]Armstrong (1972), p. 1582.

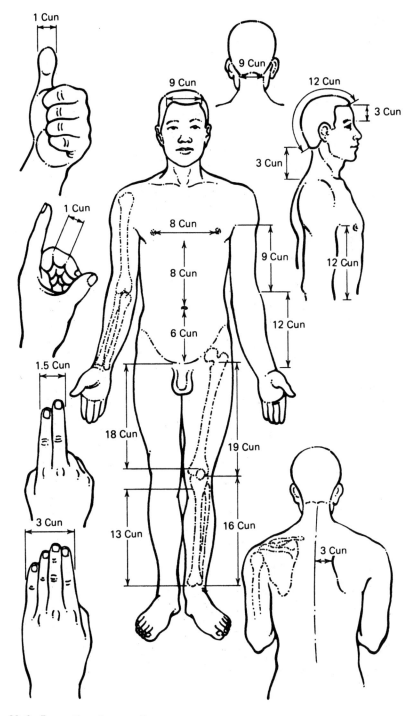

**Figure 20-9.** Proportional cun units.

TABLE 20-2.    TABLE FOR PROPORTIONAL MEASUREMENT

| Distance | Cun | Remarks |
|---|---|---|
| **Head** | | |
| Anterior hairline to posterior hairline | 12 | If hairlines are indistinguishable, measure the glabella to the process of the seventh cervical vertebra as 18 cun |
| Anterior hairline to glabella | 3 | |
| Posterior hairline to the process of the seventh cervical vertebra | 3 | |
| The hairline between the two temporal regions | 9 | Between the tips of the two mastoid processes is also measured as 9 cun |
| **Thorax & Abdomen** | | |
| Distance between the two nipples | 8 | The anterior aspect of chest is measured in accordance with intercostal space. Width of every rib is measured as 1.6 cun |
| From lower end of sternum to center of umbilicus | 8 | |
| Center of umbilicus to upper border of symphysis pubis | 5 | |
| Axillary crease to tip of eleventh rib | 12 | |
| **Back** | | |
| Medial border of scapula to midline of back | 3 | To locate points lengthwise at the back, the intervertebral space may be taken as a landmark |
| **Upper Extremities** | | |
| Transverse axiliary fold to cubital crease | 9 | Identical for lateral and medial aspects |
| Cubital crease to transverse wrist crease | 12 | |
| **Lower Extremities** | | |
| Upper level of the greater trochanter to middle of patella | 19 | Identical for anterior, posterior, and lateral aspects |
| Middle of patella to tip of lateral malleolus | 16 | |
| Upper border of symphysis pubis to upper border of epicondyle of the femur | 18 | Identical for medial aspect |
| Medial condyle of the tibia to the tip of medial malleolus | 13 | |

**TABLE 20–3.  LOCATION OF THE 20 MOST USEFUL ACUPUNCTURE POINTS**

| Acupuncture Point | Chinese Name and Meaning | Location | Indications |
|---|---|---|---|
| Urinary Bladder-40 B-40 | Wei-Chung "Commanding Middle" | At the center of the popliteal fossa | Low back pain<br>Sciatica<br>Lower extremity paralysis<br>Leg cramp<br>Disorders of hip joint and surrounding soft tissue<br>Knee joint pain, arthritis<br>Heat stroke<br>Apoplexy<br>Epilepsy<br>Acute gastroenteritis<br>Cystitis |
| Urinary Bladder-60 B-60 | Kunlun "Mountain" | Midpoint between the posterior margin of the lateral malleolus and the Achilles tendon | Lower extremity paralysis<br>Low back pain<br>Sciatica<br>Disorders of the ankle joint and surrounding soft tissue |
| Gall Bladder-20 GB-20 | Feng-chih "Wind Pond" | Midpoint of a line joining the tip of the mastoid process to the posterior midline in the groove between the trapezius and the sternoclei-domastoid | Tension headache<br>Migraine headache<br>Stiff neck<br>Dizziness<br>Vertigo<br>Common cold<br>Hypertension<br>Tinnitus |
| Gall Bladder-21 GB-21 | Chieng-ching "Shoulder Well" | Midway between C-7 and acromion process | Shoulder and back pain<br>Neck pain and rigidity<br>Upper extremity motor impairment<br>Mastisis<br>Hyperthyroidism<br>Functional uterine bleeding |
| Gall Bladder-30 GB-30 | Huan-tiao "Jumping Circle" | One third of the distance from the greater trochanter to the base of the coccyx | Hip joint pain<br>Sciatica<br>Low back pain<br>Lower extremity paralysis<br>Disorders of hip joint and surrounding soft tissue |
| Gall Bladder-34 GB-34 | Yangling Chuan "Yang Mound Spring" | Anterior to the neck of the fibula | Hemiplegia<br>Diseases of the gallbladder<br>Low back pain<br>Dizziness<br>Vertigo<br>Acid regurgitation<br>Lower extremity and knee pain |

*(cont.)*

TABLE 20–3. *(Continued)*

| Acupuncture Point | Chinese Name and Meaning | Location | Indications |
|---|---|---|---|
| Governing Vessel-26 GV-26 | Jan-chung "Middle of the Man" | One third of the distance from the inferior surface of the nose to the upper lip line | Shock<br>Heat stroke<br>Low back pain<br>Epilepsy<br>Facial paralysis |
| Large Intestines-4 LI-4 | Ho-Ku "Meeting Valley" | Between first and second metacarpals | Foreheadache<br>Toothache<br>Temporomandibular joint arthritis<br>Tonsilitis<br>Rhinitis<br>Oropharyngitis<br>Facial paralysis<br>Pain and paralysis of upper extremity<br>Hyperhydrosis<br>Goiter<br>Eye disease<br>Fever<br>Hemiplegia<br>Analgesia<br>Abdominal pain<br>Common cold—coughing<br>Amenorrhea<br>Delirium<br>Induction of labor<br>Insomnia<br>Prostration<br>Asthma<br>Anesthesia for dental work—especially for lower jaw |
| Large Intestines-11 LI-11 | Chu-chih "Crooked Pond" | Radial end of fold of fully flexed elbow | Shoulder and elbow pain<br>Paralysis of upper extremity<br>Hypertension<br>Disorders of elbow joint and surrounding soft tissue<br>Fever<br>Common cold<br>Chorea<br>Eczema<br>Neurodermatitis |
| Large Intestines-15 LI-15 | Chien-yu "Shoulder Bone" | In the depression of the acromion in the center of the deltoid muscle when the arm is abducted to 90° | Pain and impaired movement of elbow and arm<br>Disorders of shoulder joint and surrounding soft tissue |

TABLE 20–3. *(Continued)*

| Acupuncture Point | Chinese Name and Meaning | Location | Indications |
|---|---|---|---|
| Large Intestines-20 LI-20 | Ying-hsiang "Welcome Fragrance" | At the lower margin and lateral to the nostrils in the nasolabial fold | Facial paralysis<br>Rhinitis<br>Sinusitis<br>Ascariasis of bile duct |
| Liver-3 Liv-3 | Tai-chung "Too Rushy" | Between the first and second metatarsals, in a fossa, just distal to the heads | Headache<br>Dizziness<br>Epilepsy |
| Lung-7 Lu-7 | Lieh-chueh "Listing Deficiency" | Proximal to styloid process of radius | Headache<br>Neck pain<br>Cough<br>Asthma<br>Facial paralysis |
| Pericardium-6 P-6 | Nei-Kuan "Inner Gate" | Two cun above ventral wrist fold between the tendons of palmaris longus and the flexor carpi radialis | Vomiting<br>Gastralgia<br>Palpitation<br>Angina pectoris<br>Hiccough<br>Chest and costal region pain<br>Stomach pain<br>Insomnia<br>Epilepsy<br>Hysteria |
| Small Intestines-3 SI-3 | Hou-chi "Back Stream" | At the apex of the distal palmar crease on the ulnar side of a clenched fist | Neck pain and rigidity<br>Low back pain<br>Tinnitus<br>Deafness<br>Occipital headache<br>Upper extremity paralysis<br>Night sweating<br>Epilepsy<br>Malaria |
| Spleen-6 Sp-6 | San-yin-chiao "Three Ying Crossing" | Three cun above medial malleolus, just behind the posterior edge of the tibia | Insomnia<br>Barborymus<br>Abdominal distention<br>Loose stool<br>Irregular menstruation<br>Nocturnal emission<br>Impotence<br>Spermatorrhea<br>Orchitis<br>Enuresis<br>Neurasthenia<br>Frequent urination<br>Hemiplegia<br>Urine retention |

*(cont.)*

**TABLE 20-3.** (*Continued*)

| Acupuncture Point | Chinese Name and Meaning | Location | Indications |
|---|---|---|---|
| Stomach-7<br>St-7 | Hsia-Kuan "Lower Gate" | In the depression at the lower border of the zygomatic arch, anterior to the condyloid process of the mandible | Toothache<br>Facial paralysis<br>Trigeminal neuralgia<br>Temporomandibular joint arthritis |
| Stomach-36<br>St-36 | Tsu-san-li "Walk Three More Miles" | One cun distal and lateral to the tibial tuberosity | Acute and chronic gastritis<br>Nausea and vomiting<br>Functional gastrointestinal disturbances<br>Digestive tract diseases<br>Neurosis<br>Some allergies<br>Fever<br>Shock<br>Aching of hips and knees<br>Leg edema or ache<br>Hemiplegia<br>Anemia<br>Headache<br>Epilepsy<br>Lumbago<br>Heaviness of head and frontal headache<br>Acute and chronic enteritis<br>Acute pancreatitis<br>Pyloric spasm<br>Jaundice<br>Urogenital ailments<br>General weakness<br>Paralytic illness |
| Special Point #1 | Yin-tang "Seal Palace" | At the glabella, midway between the medial margins of the eyebrows | Diseases of the nose<br>Headache<br>Dizziness<br>Vertigo |
| Special Point #2 | Tai-yang "Supreme Yang" | At the temple, one cun directly posterior to the midpoint of a line joining the lateral canthus of the eye and the lateral margin of the eyebrow | Migraine<br>Trigeminal neuralgia<br>Eye diseases<br>Toothache<br>Facial paralysis |

Use one finger, usually the middle finger or the thumb, to press against the acupuncture point. Small friction-like circular movements may be used to work one's way toward deeper pressure with the ultimate objective being that of deep, constant pressure on the accurate acupuncture point. Effective treatment time ranges from one to five minutes per point per treatment, or until the patient claims relief. The author has actually heard patients say, in reference to pain, "It's going away. . . . It's going away. . . . It's gone!"

Some contraindications exist, especially for people who are not fully trained in acupuncture. Avoid using these techniques directly over contusions, scar tissue or infection, or if the patient has a serious cardiac condition. Discontinue treatment immediately if the patient appears aggravated or if no improvement is observable. Children under 7 years of age should not be treated with these techniques.

The 20 most useful acupuncture points will be used as examples to indicate the wide variety of disabilities that can be treated effectively using finger pressure to acupuncture points. Pressure application must be applied to the *exact point* or treatment will be useless.

Figure 20–9 and Table 20–2 provide an explanation of proportional cun units, based on the patient's hand measurement, not the acupuncturist's.[12] Table 20–3 provides information as to the location of these 20 points (*see also* Figs. 20–10 to 20–28 for anatomical diagrams of point locations) and the disabilities indicated that can be partially or totally relieved by pressure at these respective points.

Table 20–4 was compiled by the author using many of the references in the bibliography and with the assistance of Joseph Yao, Donald Courtial, and Dorothy McLaughlin. It is designed to provide quick, easy reference for those using this text to enable them to incorporate finger pressure into their treatment programs.

The idea should be reinforced that any or all of the massage systems described in this text may be used alone or in combination. Any massage system used depends on the responses of individual disabilities and the particular physiologic and psychologic reactions to the treatment being given, as well as the individual's response to the person providing the treatment.

---

[12]Reprinted from Academy of Traditional Chinese Medicine. (1975). *An outline of Chinese acupuncture*. Peking: Foreign Language Press, p. 6.

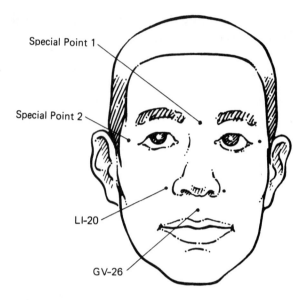

**Figure 20-10.** Acupuncture points on the face.

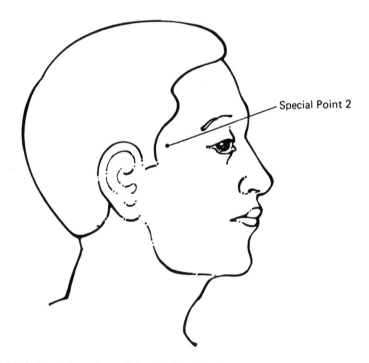

**Figure 20-11.** Lateral view of special point 2 on the face.

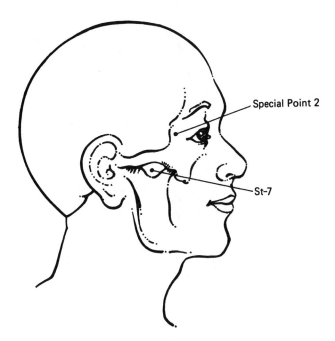

**Figure 20-12.** Lateral view of special points 2 and St. 7 on the face.

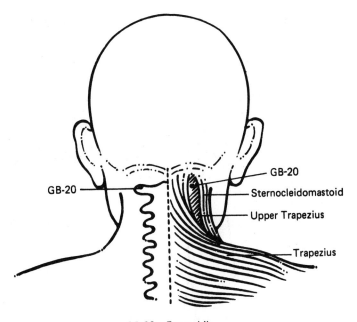

GB-20— Feng-chih

**Figure 20-13.** Acupuncture point GB-20 Feng-chih.

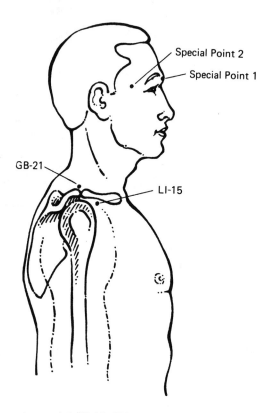

**Figure 20-14.** Acupuncture point GB-21, Chien-ching, and LI-15 Chien-yu, lateral view.

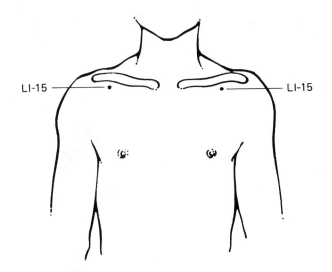

**Figure 20-15.** Acupuncture point LI-15 Chien-yu, frontal view.

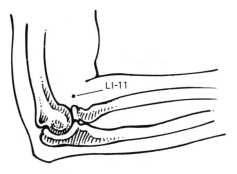

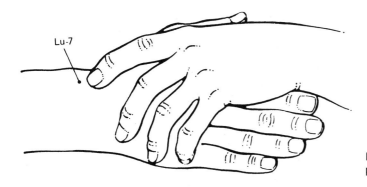

Figure 20-16. Acupuncture point LI-11 Chu-chih.

Figure 20-17. Acupuncture point LU-7 Lieh-chueh.

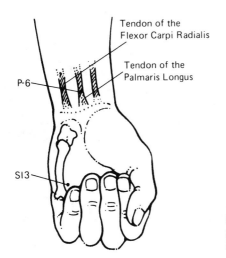

Figure 20-18. Acupuncture point P-6 Nei-Kuan and S-13 Hou-chi.

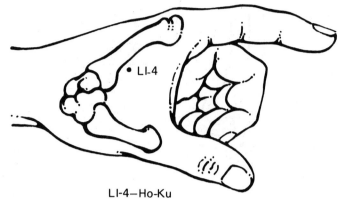

LI-4–Ho-Ku

**Figure 20-19.** Acupuncture point LI-4 Ho-Ku.

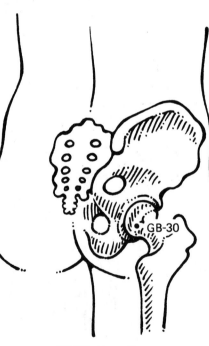

GB-30–Huan-Tiao

**Figure 20-20.** Acupuncture point GB-30 Huan-tiao, lateral view.

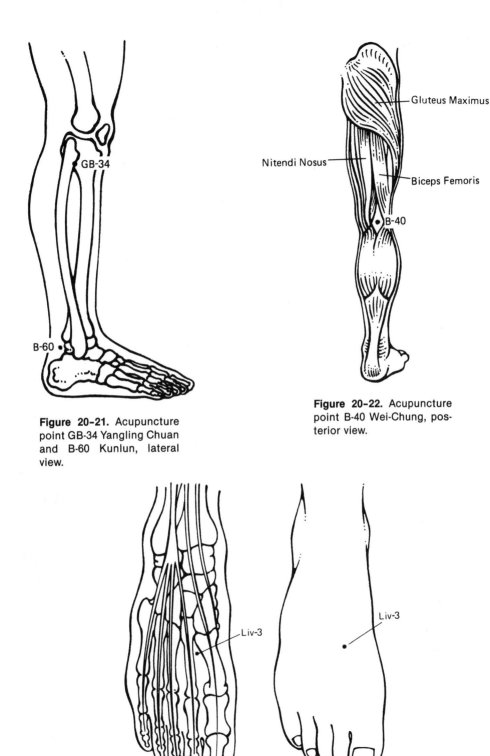

**Figure 20-21.** Acupuncture point GB-34 Yangling Chuan and B-60 Kunlun, lateral view.

GB-34

B-60

Gluteus Maximus

Nitendi Nosus

Biceps Femoris

B-40

**Figure 20-22.** Acupuncture point B-40 Wei-Chung, posterior view.

Liv-3

Liv-3

**Figure 20-23.** Acupuncture point Liv-3 Tai-chung, frontal foot view.

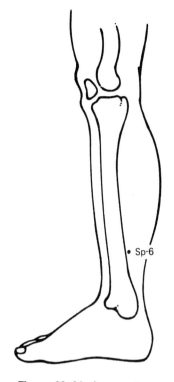

**Figure 20-24.** Acupuncture point SP-6 San-yin-chiao, lateral view.

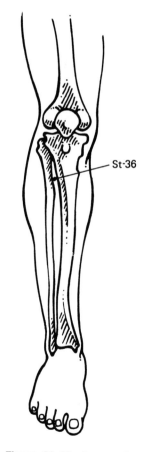

**Figure 20-25.** Acupuncture point St.-36 Tsu-san-li, frontal view.

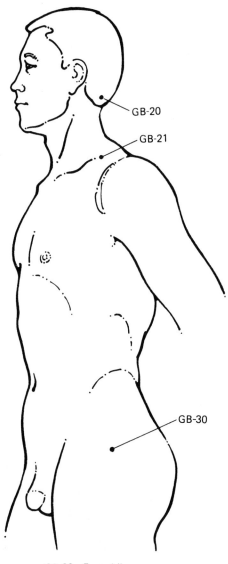

GB-20— Feng-chih
GB-21—Chien-ching
GB-30—Huan-tiao

**Figure 20-26.** Lateral view GB-20 Feng-chih, GB-21 Chien-ching, GB-30 Huan-tiao.

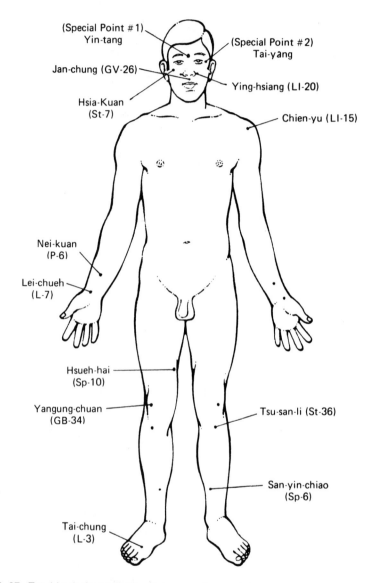

**Figure 20–27.** Total body frontal view of acupuncture points.

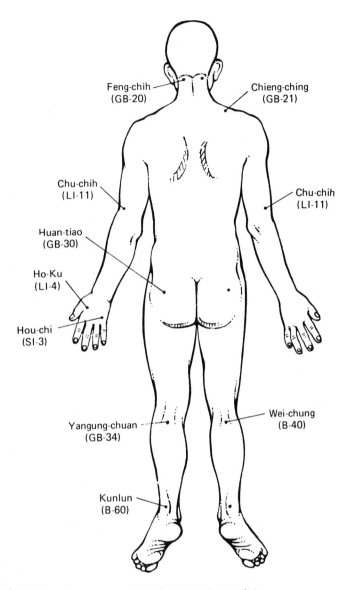

**Figure 20-28.** Total body posterior view of acupuncture points.

**TABLE 20-4. SOME COMBINATIONS OF THESE 20 POINTS FOR VARIOUS DISORDERS**

### Headache

**Frontal—"Heaviness of Head"**
Large Intestine 4
Special Point #1
Stomach 36

**Vertical headache**
Urinary Bladder 60

**Tension headache**
Gall Bladder 20
Gall Bladder 21
Large Intestine 4
Liver 3
Special Point #1

**Migraine headache**
Gall Bladder 20
Gall Bladder 36
Large Intestine 4
Liver 3
Special Point #2
Stomach 36

**Sinus headache—Chronic**
Rhinitis
Gall Bladder 20
Large Intestine 4
Large Intestine 20
Lung 7
Special Point #1

**Diseases of the head, face, trunk, and internal organs**
Gall Bladder 34
Large Intestine 4
Small Intestine 3
Stomach 36

**Temporomandibular headache**
Gall Bladder 20
Special Point #2

**Occipital headache**
Gall Bladder 20
Gall Bladder 21
Liver 3
Small Intestine 3
Urinary Bladder 60

**Trigeminal nerve—Facial**
Paralysis
Governing Vessel 26
Large Intestine 4
Large Intestine 20
Lung 7
Special Point #2
Stomach 7

**Generalized headache**
Large Intestine 4
Special Point #1

**From malfunction of the liver**
Large Intestine 4
Large Intestine 11
Urinary Bladder 40

**Neck disorders**
Gall Bladder 20
Gall Bladder 21
Lung 7

### Disorders of the Upper Extremity

**Shoulder disorders**
Gall Bladder 21
Large Intestine 11

**Elbow disorders**
Gall Bladder 21
Large Intestine 4
Large Intestine 11
Large Intestine 15
Small Intestine 3

### Disorders of the Trunk and Lower Extremity

**Low back pain**
Gall Bladder 34
Governing Vessel 34
Small Intestine 3
Urinary Bladder 40
Urinary Bladder 60

**Sciatica**
Gall Bladder 30
Gall Bladder 34
Urinary Bladder 40
Urinary Bladder 60

TABLE 20-4.    *(Continued)*

## Disorders of the Trunk and Lower Extremity *(cont.)*

**Lower extremity involvement—**
**pain, paralysis, fatigue**
Gall Bladder 30
Gall Bladder 34
Stomach 36
Urinary Bladder 40
Urinary Bladder 60

**Disorders of hip joint and**
**surrounding soft tissue**
Gall Bladder 30
Gall Bladder 34
Urinary Bladder 40

**Knee pain**
Gall Bladder 34
Large Intestine 4
Stomach 36
Spleen 6
Urinary Bladder 40

**Disorders of the ankle joint and**
**surrounding soft tissue**
Gall Bladder 34
Urinary Bladder 60

**Muscular dysfunction of the feet**
Spleen 6
Stomach 36

## Systemic Disorders

**Common cold**
Gall Bladder 20
Large Intestine 4
Large Intestine 20
Lung 7
Special Point #1

**Cough**
Lung 7
Spleen 6

**Dizziness**
Gall Bladder 20
Gall Bladder 34
Liver 3
Special Point #1

**Epilepsy**
Gall Bladder 34
Small Intestine 3

**Fever**
Large Intestine 4
Large Intestine 11

**Heat stroke**
Governing Vessel 26
Urinary Bladder 40

**Hemiplegia**
Gall Bladder 34
Large Intestine 4
Spleen 6

**Hypertension**
Gall Bladder 20
Large Intestine 4
Large Intestine 11
Stomach 36
Spleen 6

**Impotence**
Stomach 36
Spleen 6

**Insomnia**
Pericardium 6
Spleen 6

**Irregular menses**
Gall Bladder 21
Large Intestine 4
Spleen 6
Stomach 36

**Morning sickness**
Pericardium 6
Stomach 36

**Nausea**
Pericardium 6
Stomach 36

**Shock**
Pericardium 6
Stomach 36

**Tinnitus**
Gall Bladder 20
Small Intestine 3

**Toothache**
Large Intestine 4
Large Intestine 20
Lung 7
Special Point #2
Stomach 7

**Vertigo**
Gall Bladder 20
Gall Bladder 34
Special Point #1

## SUMMARY

Since 1958, Western medicine's interest in the effectiveness of acupuncture has increased. Both Eastern and Western medicine are actively involved in research to explain physiologically or psychologically how acupuncture accomplishes anesthesia and even euphoria. The reasons for its effectiveness become clearer as research continues in the methods of pain relief and endorphins (*see* Endogenous Morphine, Chapter 6).

This chapter presents a brief history of acupuncture as well as a discussion of the Oriental theories related to meridians. The discussion of 20 selected points provides the reader with general knowledge of the most commonly used points and the disabilities that can effectively benefit from finger pressure on specific points. The bibliography provides complete information related to hundreds of other acupuncture points. The reader should pursue the literature for more complete information.

# —21

# Jin Shin Do

Jasmine Ellen Wolf with Iona Marsaa Teeguarden

Jin Shin Do is a relatively new method of releasing muscular tension and stress by applying deepening finger pressure to combinations of specific points on the body. These points, called *acupoints,* are highly energized spots along the meridians—pathways of energy associated with body organs (see Chapter 19 for descriptions and diagrams of meridians).

Jin Shin Do, which may be translated as *the way of the compassionate spirit,* is a modern synthesis of traditional Oriental acupressure–acupuncture theory and techniques, breathing exercises, Taoist philosophy, and modern psychology. Iona Marsaa Teeguarden, who lives in California, researched various acupressure techniques in the 1970s and, in 1978, wrote *Acupressure Way of Health.*[1] This book describes the basic principles behind her synthesis, which she calls *Jin Shin Do.* In the ensuing years, she added psychology to this synthesis, as described in *The Joy of Feeling: Bodymind℠ Acupressure.*[2] In 1982, Teeguarden founded the Jin Shin Do Foundation® to train and network authorized teachers of this method.[3]

## ARMORED ACUPOINTS

Applying simple, direct finger pressure to acupoints helps to release tension and reduce physical and emotional stress. In Oriental terms, these acu-

---

[1] Iona Teeguarden. (1978). *Acupressure way of health: Jin Shin Do.* New York: Japan Publications/Harper & Row.

[2] Iona Teeguarden. (1987). *Joy of feeling: Bodymind℠ acupressure.* New York: Japan Publications/Harper & Row.

[3] For more information and a directory of authorized teachers, contact the Jin Shin Do Foundation®, P.O. Box 1800, Idyllwild, CA 92349, (714)659–5550.

points are places along the meridians where the life force energy comes close to the surface of the body. In Western terms, they are places of high electrical conductivity or low electrical resistance, compared to the surrounding area.

When a person experiences stress due to environmental, social, emotional, or physical stimuli, tension (and energy) tends to collect at some of these points. If the tension is not released, the tension acts like a record of the stressful experience or situation. Future incidents may remind the person unconsciously of the original stress or trauma. For instance, a child who is physically or emotionally abused may tighten certain body parts to numb the pain or to suppress tears or shouts in order to avoid further punishment. Stress may be induced years later by the replication of smells, sights, or sounds experienced during these early traumatic events, but the person may not be aware of why she or he is feeling more stressed in these situations. Meanwhile, the points of tension (for example, in the neck, shoulders, or back) become tighter and tighter and feel increasingly hard to the touch. This chronic tension that is called *armoring*, is often located on the acupoints. An armored area is shown diagrammatically in Figure 21–1.

Because armored points contain a psychologic history, sometimes suppressed emotions or old defensive attitudes will surface to conscious awareness during the release of these points. Jin Shin Do practitioners are trained to empathize with and help people go through such emotional releases as well as to help release physical stress and refer people to psychotherapists and doctors when necessary. Jin Shin Do is not a medical treatment. It is a transformational process, involving consciousness in restoring balance to body, mind, emotions, and spirit.

Jin Shin Do is a gentle way to release muscular tension and armoring. The practitioner starts with light pressure and penetrates deeper when "invited in" by the client. The practitioner stays on the point for a relatively long time and is, therefore, able to work deeply. While one hand is holding

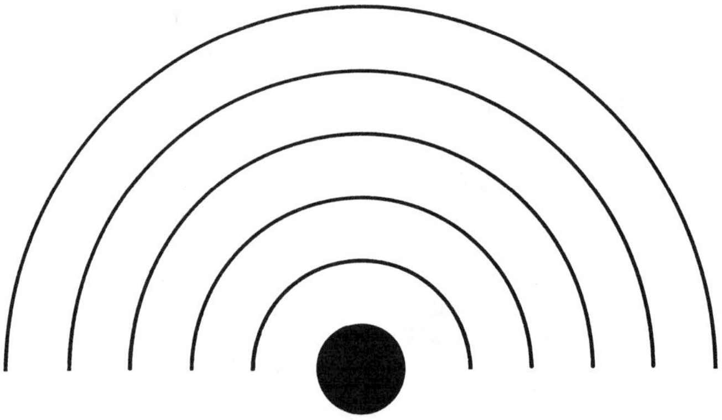

**Figure 21-1.** An area of armoring. Subsequent layers of tension may be related to subsequent events that remind the person of the original stressor.

Original Tension
(trauma)

a tense place, the other hand holds a series of other points, which helps release the tension and balance the body energy, enabling the release to be more pleasurable and more effective. Even so, it is rarely possible or advisable to release all the tension from an armored area in a single session. People are usually not able to handle too revolutionary a change at once, just as they are not prepared to confront their entire psychologic history too quickly.

Trained practitioners help people pay attention to the sensations and feelings that accompany release or armoring, and to learn and grow from the emotions and imagery that arise. Release is often accompanied by deep relaxation, or occasionally by tingling and trembling, crying or shouting. Sometimes, the process is peaceful and internal, perhaps with the recipient falling asleep during the session. Often the release is followed by a new resolution, on a conscious or unconscious level, and a renewed ability to live joyfully.

## STRANGE FLOWS

Ancient Oriental philosophers believed that the body is a microcosm of what is on earth and in the universe. These philosophers observed that when rivers overflow, the excess water forms channels and flows to a river that lacks water. Therefore, these philosophers postulated that when a meridian becomes excessively filled with energy, the excess collects in channels and is redistributed to deficient meridians. These channels are called *strange flows* or *wondrous channels*.

Unlike the flow through the meridians, energy does not flow continuously through the strange flows, but only when the energy is unevenly distributed among the meridians. The strange flows (with the exception of the great central channel [GCC]) have no acupoints of their own: all their points are on major meridians.

If the strange flows were free from blockage, the body would maintain harmony and balance through the meridians. However, the strange flows are also subject to armoring and blockages. A Jin Shin Do practitioner can balance the meridians without assessing them by releasing the strange flows.

There are four pairs of strange flows— the Yin and Yang great regulator channels (GRC), the Yin and Yang great bridge channel (GBC), the belt channel (BC) and penetrating channel (PC), and the conception vessel (CV) and governing vessel (GV). The CV and GV combined are the GCC. Release of the GCC (which is shown in a simplified form in Fig. 21–2) is good for people with minor spinal or constitutional disorders (check with their doctor or chiropractor first) and it is used to balance the reproductive system, particularly in women. It is also effective for helping psychic energy flow. The Yin and Yang GRCs are used for people who are suffering from shoulder or neck tension or from nervous tension. The Yin and Yang GBCs are chosen for people with back tension. They also help increase a person's energy and are

Hold this point throughout the back release with your right hand (Steps 1 through 4)

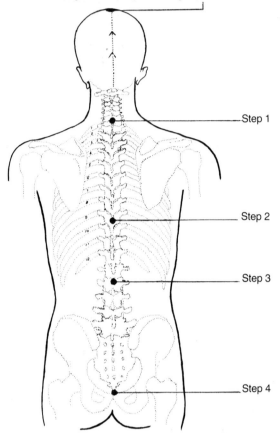

Step 1

Step 2

Step 3

Step 4

**Figure 21-2A&B.** The great central channel. **A.** The back release (the governing vessel). The practitioner should sit on the left. The receiver always lies face up. (Figure **A** is shown face down so the practitioner can locate the back points used in this release.) When pressing points on a person's back, the practitioner reaches under the receiver's back and uses the person's weight to help regulate the pressure. When pressing any back points in this release, the finger that is pressing always points straight up toward the ceiling. Step 1. Place either one finger or the palm of your right hand over the top of the receiver's head. Your right hand or finger will stay here throughout the next four steps. Place one finger of your left hand between the seventh cervical and first thoracic vertebrae. It is important that you press all points on the great central channel *gently*. Step 2. Place one finger of your left hand between the ninth and tenth thoracic vertebrae. Step 3. Place one finger of your left hand between the second and third lumbar vertebrae. Step 4. Place the palm of your left hand against the receiver's coccyx.

the channels that are traditionally released on athletes. The PC and BC help release the abdominal and low back areas and strengthen the sexual energy and organs.[4]

---

[4]Detailed instructions for releasing all the strange flows can be found in Teeguarden (1978).

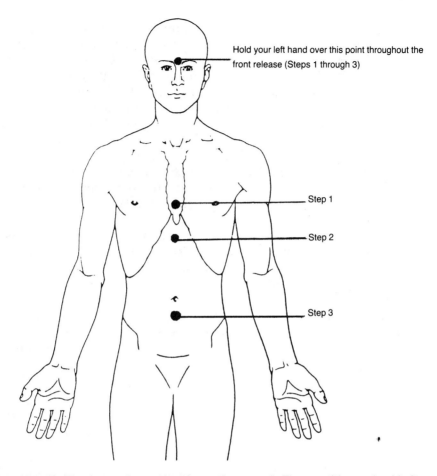

**Figure 21-2B.** The front release (the conception vessel). The practitioner should sit on the right. The receiver lies face up. Step 1. Place the palm of your left hand over the receiver's "third eye" (just above and between the eyes). Your left hand will stay on the third eye throughout the next three steps. Place either one finger or the palm of your right hand over the midpoint between the receiver's nipples and press. Step 2. Place you right palm over the receiver's solar plexus and press. Step 3. Place your right palm over the receiver's lower abdomen (hara).

## ASSESSMENT OF MERIDIANS

Although the strange flows can be released without assessment, more accurate meridian balancing requires assessment of the energy flow. Theoretically, if the energy were flowing freely, our bodies would be working perfectly, and we would not experience physical, mental, emotional, or spiritual tension or dis-ease. In Jin Shin Do, releasing tension and enhancing bodymind well-being involves the assessment of which meridians and flows are imbalanced, as well as of which parts of the body are most tense or armored.

The emphasis is on energetic imbalance and muscular relaxation, not on symptoms. For example, in the case of the common cold, there may be imbalance of the lung meridian, which would be the most obvious possibility. Nevertheless, assessment of the meridians may indicate that the problem is imbalance of the triple-warmer meridian (which pertains to the maintenance of homeostasis of body temperature and energy production). Or, the problem may have begun with a liver meridian imbalance; perhaps the patient is having a problem with toxicity (perhaps toxic anger). Or, there may be a kidney meridian imbalance, indicating that the patient's reserve energy is drained (perhaps due to chronic stress). People with imbalanced gall bladder meridians may be so tortured by decision making that they make themselves sick. Wherever the imbalance starts, if it is not corrected, other meridians may gradually be affected in a domino-like fashion. According to the traditional theory behind Jin Shin Do, the bodymind is one whole, and problems in one part of the system will affect other parts.

It is important to note that we are assessing meridians, *not* organs. A meridian can be out of balance, and yet the person can be physically healthy. For instance, a heart meridian imbalance is much more likely to indicate heartache or difficulty with intimate relationships than physical heart problems. Meridians are symbols, and as such they have many meanings. In Oriental theory, the meridians are associated not only with body organs, but also with specific senses, colors, expressions, emotions, tastes, and activities. An imbalance in a meridian may be reflected as either an excess or a deficiency in these areas. There are seasons and times of day when the energy is strongest in each meridian. During a meridian's associated "time" or "season" strengths and weaknesses of the meridian are accented.

The twelve "organ meridians" fall within the five categories of metal, earth, fire, water, and wood. These elements are symbols for five energic tendencies, or for five aspects of the bodymind whole.

Some key associations for each meridian are listed in Table 21–1. This is not a definitive list, but these functional relationships will give the reader some idea of the essentially holistic concepts of acupressure theory.

There are several ways to assess the related meridians, including pulse reading and assessing the abdomen (hara) and back. Another method is to observe and ask questions, designing the questions to find out information such as that given in Table 21–1. Let us consider some examples.

Which sense is most important or works best for the patient? Which sense is weak? If a patient has a problem with a sense organ, weakness in the corresponding meridian may be indicated. For example, depending extensively on the sense of sight and not being able to smell very well may indicate both metal and wood imbalance. Similarly, too much or too little of a body liquid could indicate an imbalance. For instance, if a person creates too much mucus or too little there may be an imbalance in the metal element—either the lung or large intestine meridian.

**TABLE 21-1.   QUALITIES OF THE FIVE ELEMENTS**

| Element: | Metal | Earth | Fire | Water | Wood |
|---|---|---|---|---|---|
| Yin | Lung | Spleen | Heart & pericardium | Kidney | Liver |
| Yang | Large intestine | Stomach | Triple warmer & small intestine | Bladder | Gall bladder |
| Sense | Smell | Taste | Speech | Hearing | Sight |
| Sense organ | Nose | Mouth, lips | Tongue | Ears | Eyes |
| Liquid | Mucus | Saliva | Sweat | Urine | Tears |
| Color | White | Yellow | Red | Blue, black | Green |
| Expression | Weeping | Singing | Laughing | Groaning | Shouting |
| Extreme emotion | Grief, anxiety | Worry, reminiscence | Shock, overjoy | Fear | Anger |
| Balanced emotion | Openness, receptivity | Sympathy, empathy | Joy, compassion | Resolution, trust, motivation | Assertion |
| Taste | Pungent, spicy | Sweet | Bitter, burned | Salty | Sour |
| Season | Fall | Indian summer | Summer | Winter | Spring |
| Related activity | Letting go | Mental activity | Inspiration & intimacy | Willpower & vitality | Planning & decision making |
| Times | Lung, 3–5 AM | Stomach, 7–9 AM | Heart, 11 AM–1 PM | Bladder, 3–5 PM | Gall bladder, 11 PM–1AM |
| | Large intestine, 5–7 AM | Spleen, 9–11 AM | Small intestine, 1–3 PM | Kidney, 5–7 PM | Pericardium, 7–9 PM Triple warmer 9–11 PM |

Look at the colors a person wears and the hue of the person's face. For instance, asthmatics are often very white, indicating a lung meridian imbalance. People with metal imbalances may love white or hate it. Listen to the patient. Some people have voices that sing (earth) and others are always shouting (wood imbalance). Some people giggle at inappropriate times, for example, when they talk about having been hurt (fire imbalance).

Which emotions cause problems? Some people are so sympathetic that they are swallowed by other people's sorrows, whereas others are unable to feel or express their sympathy. In both cases there is likely to be an earth imbalance.

Times of day when a person feels tired or uncomfortable can help point out imbalances. A person who feels tired at 2 PM probably has a small intestine meridian imbalance since the small intestine "time" is from 1 to 3 PM.

The way people express themselves also reveals imbalances. For example, intellectuals tend to have earth imbalances as do people who scorn the intellect, whereas a fear of intimacy suggests a fire imbalance.

Assessment is nonjudgmental. In the Oriental frame of mind, nothing is good or bad. In Western society, anger is often considered "bad." Notice that anger is a wood element quality along with spring and green. When it flows smoothly, anger is an honest, spontaneous emotion from the heart, and such anger is often felt toward a loved one or someone considered important. Healthy anger can be a renewal because it can clear away the debris in a relationship. On the other hand, stifled anger festers and becomes toxic, and like explosive anger it suggests a wood imbalance.

Another way to assess meridians in the body is to touch the *associated points* and determine whether they are tense or sore. These points are located on the back along the two bladder meridian lines that are on the edges of the erector spinae. On these lines, the points parallel to the spaces between the vertebrae correspond to specific meridians (Fig. 21–3). If the tension is mostly on the medial edge of the erector spinae, then the problem is short term or in the early stages of development, and if the tension is on the outer edge of the muscle then the imbalance is chronic. For instance, the points on these lines that are next to the discs between the third and fourth thoracic vertebrae are associated with the lung meridian. If the lung meridian is weak, then the third or fourth thoracic vertebrae may be out of alignment or the area around one or both of the lung associated points may be tense or lifeless, colorless or excessively colored, hot or cold, or may have some other unusual quality. These points may be sore when touched or may be so armored that they are numb. There may also be muscle spasms in this area.

In Jin Shin Do, the practitioner first chooses a meridian to work with and then chooses a point on that meridian needing to be released. For instance, in working with the lung meridian, a point called #30 is a good choice for a *local point,* that is, a point that is the site of the problem or of excessive tension. This point is held for about 2 min while at least two other points on the lung meridian are pressed, one after the other. These points are called *distal points* because they are distant from the site of the problem, but they facilitate deeper release of the local point. Because of the connection created between the two stimulated points, both points are released more efficiently than they would be if only one point were held at a time. It is necessary to study Jin Shin Do with a trained practitioner in order to know how to effectively release the meridians, but Figure 21–4 provides an example of how you might work with the lung meridian.

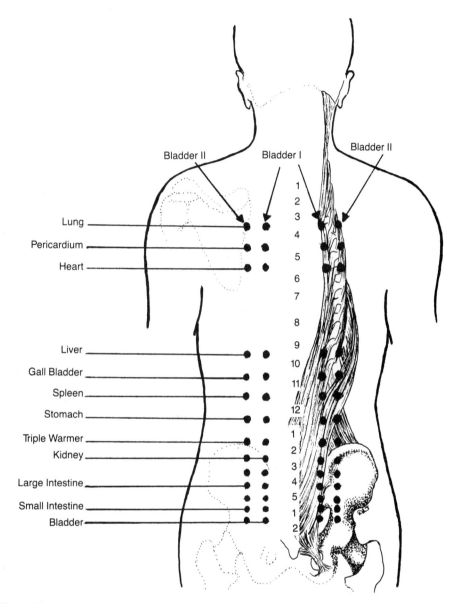

**Figure 21-3.** Meridian assessment.

## BODY SEGMENTS

Jin Shin Do practitioners also work in terms of *body segments*. These are groups of muscles that are functionally related and that work together to make expressive movements and gestures. For example, if you grit your

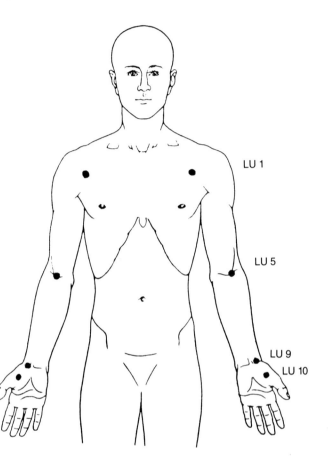

**Figure 21-4.** Lung meridian. Some release points on the lung meridian. While one hand holds the local point known as #30 in Jin Shin Do numbering (called Lung 1 in acupuncture), the other could hold several distal points along the Lung meridian, such as point #36 (Lung 10 in acupuncture) at the base of the wrist.

LU 1

LU 5

LU 9

LU 10

teeth you can feel the back of your neck tensing. Therefore, these areas are part of the same segment. For this reason it is impossible to fully release the neck until tension is released from the jaw. The major body segments are shown in Figure 21–5.

Determining which segments are tense also helps the practitioner understand a patient's emotional conflicts. The chest, for instance, reveals how we do or do not let our feelings flow. People with inflated chests are likely to have a macho facade and to act stronger than they really are. One way to correlate the segments and emotions is to think of clichés associated with the tight segments, such as "carrying the weight of the world on my shoulders," or "I can't stomach the situation." Table 21–2 provides examples of emotional correlations with the major body segments.

Usually, all the segments need some release. In Jin Shin Do, the usual procedure is to release the segments from the top down, first freeing the areas related to self-expression. Then, when energy is released in the lower

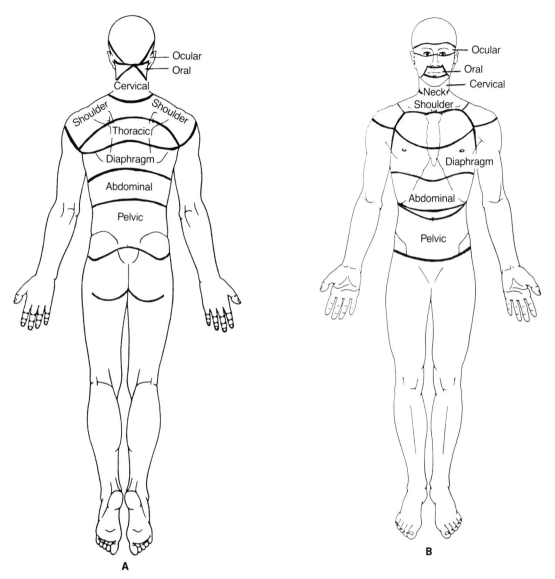

**Figure 21-5A&B.** Major body segments.

segments, it does not get stuck when it flows up the back along the strange flows. When the upper segments are free, the person is more able to release stagnated energy through vocal expression. All Jin Shin Do sessions end with a neck release to be sure that this often tense area is relaxed—and because the neck release is very pleasurable (Fig. 21–6).

**TABLE 21-2. EMOTIONAL ASSOCIATIONS WITH THE BODY SEGMENTS**

| Body Segment | Emotional Association |
| --- | --- |
| Ocular and oral | Expression<br>Rational thinking |
| Neck | Division between rational and feeling parts of the body<br>Choking down feelings<br>Difficulty in expression |
| Shoulder | Responsibility<br>Judgment (including self-judgment) |
| Chest | Restricting the flow of our emotions<br>Restricting breathing is the way to restrict feelings<br>In the heart segment we experience appreciation and love as well as the loss of love (heartache or heartbreak) |
| Diaphragm and abdominal | Emotional and intrapersonal power<br>Fear of losing oneself to one's feelings<br>In this society we are told to hold our stomachs in, an area related to our personal power and gut feelings. In the Orient, by contrast, the ideal is a relaxed and slightly large stomach |
| Pelvic | This is the segment we cannot talk about—sex and elimination<br>Fear of our primary survival needs or of losing control to our primal self |

*More information on the segments is found in Iona Marsaa Teeguarden. (1987). The joy of feeling: Bodymind acupressure. New York: Japan Publications/Harper & Row.*

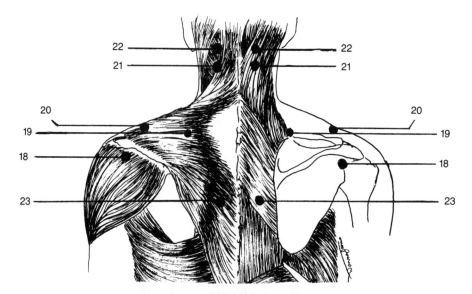

**Figure 21-6.** Neck and shoulder release. The recipient lies on his or her back; the operator sits at the head. Place hands under the shoulders and use one finger of each hand to hold both 23s until they release. Then hold both 18s until they release. Then with the fingers over the shoulders, press the thumbs into the 19s until they release, followed by thumb pressure to the 20s until they release. Next press the 21s with the fingers. The operator finishes by pulling the occipital ridge toward him or her, pressing the 22s until they release.

## HOW TO GIVE JIN SHIN DO SESSIONS

It is very simple to learn to use Jin Shin Do at a basic level for self-help and to help family and friends. After studying the 20-hour basic course, students are able to give many types of full sessions by following various release examples, or by creating their own combination of points. The only motion in a Jin Shin Do session is pressing points and holding them. The point most requiring release is called the local point. The local point is held continuously while at least two distal points are held, one after the other. The distal points are chosen by their relationship to the local point. Usually, the two points are in the same segment, on the same meridian, or on the same strange flow.

A pressure point is held by pressing a finger against the point firmly, but not so deeply that the recipient cannot relax. As the point releases, the practitioner's finger will automatically sink deeper into the point. The points are held for an average of one to two min or until the following occurs:

1. The practitioner feels the muscle relax to a significant degree.
2. The practitioner feels a pulsation or an increase in pulsation. (It might take practice to be able to feel this.)
3. The recipient feels a decrease (or sometimes, first, an increase) in sensitivity.

## BENEFITS OF JIN SHIN DO

### Psychologic Benefits

Much dis-ease is associated with destructive thought patterns often created in early childhood as an adaptive mechanism.

Now a woman in her 30s, Andrea was taught by her father not to be an "overemotional wimp." When Andrea first came to the author for treatment, she had severe asthma and had taken medication nightly for the past 12 years. The medication was no longer of value. Andrea told the author that she never cried and that she held her anger inside until she exploded uncontrollably. When she was angry she would grit her teeth, sometimes to the point of breaking them. Andrea had a very white complexion and assessment indicated that the energy in her lung meridian was excessive. The author used the lung meridian release in the *Jin Shin Do Handbook* (2nd ed.),[5] which includes #30 (lung 1), several other lung meridian points, and other points on the chest segment.

During the sessions, Andrea explained that her asthma had been very severe for the past month. Asked if anything significant had happened in

---

[5]Iona Marsaa Teeguarden. (1981). *Jin Shin Do handbook* (2nd ed.). Idyllwild, CA: Jin Shin Do Foundation, p. 8.

her life a month ago, Andrea explained that her aunt had died, but true to her training, she had not cried. When the author explained that Andrea might be choking on her own emotions, Andrea agreed to let herself cry rather than suffocate herself. By the end of the session, her complexion was red. She did not need to use her medication once for as long as the author kept in contact with her, which was 9 mo. Although hiding her emotions was destructive, this behavior was originally adaptive, for it had helped Andrea to win her father's love.

One purpose of Jin Shin Do is to help people become aware of the bodymind connection. Very often, people believe their body is "doing it to them." Our bodies are not separate entities that are giving us pain. When we learn to look for the cause of our pain within ourselves, we can accept it and then be ready to use our minds to transform our health. It is important to learn from our tensions rather than judge them. The Chinese word for crisis is composed of two characters—"danger" and "opportunity." It is the practitioner's job to help the patient become aware of the opportunity for growth that is contained in tensions, pains, or other health crises. Patients can use this knowledge as they wish. Some people need their diseases.

Jin Shin Do practitioners are not magical healers. They are more like midwives to a patient's self-healing. The most a practitioner can do is point out the deterrents to a person's health and help facilitate their release. People can only heal themselves. (As noted earlier, they occasionally need the help of doctors, physical therapists, or psychotherapists to do so.)

In Jin Shin Do practice, health is seen as a balance of the vital energies and of the bodymind–spirit. Health is not an achievement to be maintained, but a continual process that includes growth and knowledge of ourselves and the world.

## Physical Benefits of Jin Shin Do

Because both the length and depth of pressure are paced to the receiver's needs, Jin Shin Do helps provide gentle and deep release of tensions, as well as reduction of stress. As Jin Shin Do involves no movement, it is excellent for people who cannot be moved or who must be worked in a specific position. Although only a small area is touched, muscles and meridians are affected all over the body. Jin Shin Do is, therefore, effective in conditions that cannot be touched. For example, a practitioner could not work directly on an injured disc, but could help the surrounding muscles to relax. In such cases, the practitioner must always work with the permission of a chiropractor or a doctor.

Jin Shin Do is excellent to use just before a chiropractic adjustment because the adjustment is likely to be easier and to last.

Project PRES (Physical Response Education System) in Santa Cruz, Calif, has been experimenting with the effects of weekly Jin Shin Do sessions on handicapped children. The research has demonstrated many benefits to these children including improvement in learning and decrease in allergies, seizures, bedwetting, constipation, night coughing, lung congestion, ear infections, runny noses, nosebleeds, skin conditions, and weight problems. The researchers reported that children were less hyperactive, less angry, and happier. One child who had never talked began to talk in three-word sentences. Another child made a gain of almost two grade levels in language development.[6] This study suggests that the use of Jin Shin Do with normal children might be of great benefit.

## SUMMARY

Jin Shin Do is a form of acupressure that works by releasing two points simultaneously. Practitioners release body segments, meridians, or strange flows (channels to balance the meridians). Because the entire body is connected, the effects of Jin Shin Do are often felt in areas that the practitioner has not touched. The practitioner paces the depth and length of pressure to the receiver's needs. Jin Shin Do practitioners also help their patients understand how their thoughts and attitudes may be related to their physical imbalances. Occasionally, the effects of Jin Shin Do are not felt for the first one or two sessions. However, it often lasts a lifetime.

---

[6]Iona Marsaa Teeguarden. (1985, August). Acupressure in the classroom. *East West Journal, 15,* 22.

# 22

# Shiatsu: An Overview

Pauline E. Sasaki

## SHIATSU AND ITS HISTORY

Humankind has always recognized that the hand can contribute powerfully to the healing process. No one has to be told that rubbing the eyes or the scalp helps to soothe the pain of a headache, and even in Western medicine, the role of the physical therapist has come to be widely accepted. In Japan, however, the use of the hand as a therapeutic tool has a time-honored history and a deep philosophical foundation.

The Japanese art of *Shiatsu* (literally, *shi* [finger] + *atsu* [pressure]) is a system for healing and health maintenance that has evolved over the course of thousands of years. Practiced informally since at least 200 BC, Shiatsu was systematized in the early 1900s and became accepted as a form of therapy widely practiced to this day.

Shiatsu derives both from the ancient healing art of acupuncture and from the traditional form of Japanese massage, *Anma*. In Japan, Anma was originally considered the equivalent of Chinese acupuncture as the method one studied to treat the human body in illness. It was recognized to have bona fide therapeutic benefits up until the end of the Tokugawa period in the eighteenth century.[1] Because this was a peaceful period in Japan's his-

---

[1]Shizuto Masunaga. (1983). *Keiraku to Shiatsu* (In Japanese). Yokosuka: Ido-No-Nihonsha, p. 1.

tory, intellectual inclinations flourished. Simultaneously, however, society became overly enamored of the pleasures and luxuries of life, with the result that Anma was reduced to being merely an instrument of psychologic and sexual pleasure. Anma as it was practiced had discarded the historic foundations that had legitimized it as a therapeutic system.

Ultimately, Shiatsu developed apart from Anma as a therapeutic discipline based once again on its original theory. In the meantime, prior to World War II, Anma became a major employer of the blind in Japan. During the American occupation of Japan when MacArthur was considering outlawing both Anma and Shiatsu (due to erroneous information that they had sexual connotations), the blind of Japan appealed to Helen Keller in America to intercede on their behalf. Their appeal was successful and Shiatsu and Anma were permitted to be practiced.[2] Eventually, this approval led to a formal school of Shiatsu, the Nippon Shiatsu School, established by Tokujiro Namikoshi in the late 1940s. Since then, Shiatsu has become a popular medical therapy that is recognized and licensed by the government.

## BASIC CONCEPTS OF SHIATSU

To understand Shiatsu, one must first understand some of the basic concepts shared by acupuncture, Shiatsu, and the Eastern healing arts in general.

The basic tenets of Eastern medicine can be traced back to China at a time between the second and third centuries BC, when in the Yellow Emperor's *Classic of Internal Medicine* a system of energy channels called *meridians* was described (*see also* Chapter 16).[3] This perception of the body as a system of meridians formed at a time when the prevailing religion forbade any type of surgical intrusion into the human body. Denied access to procedures that would reveal the structure and functions of the human body, the Chinese developed a practical metaphor for the anatomy and physiology of the body through observation and intuition. They conceptualized the body as a living, dynamic entity subject to the influences of an underlying network of energy pathways. Thus, meridians represented the energetic, as opposed to the anatomic, structure of the body.

This emphasis on energy rather than anatomy is perhaps the fundamental difference between Eastern and Western medicine. When the body is analyzed anatomically, it appears as a collection of separate parts that exist whether the owner of the body is alive or dead. Examined energetically, however, the body appears to function as the result of a dynamic life force (referred to as *Ki*) that serves as the common link among all the body's tissues and organs. Ki ties together all bodily structures and functions so that

---

[2]Wataru Ohashi. (1976). *Do-it yourself Shiatsu.* New York: Dutton, p. 10.
[3]Yoshiaki Omura. (1982). *Acupuncture medicine.* Tokyo: Japan Publications, p. 13.

they operate as a single entity. To the Easterner, the organs are not sufficient to sustain life unless the vital force Ki is also present to keep the organs functional and properly interrelated. Furthermore, since Ki represents the essence of life, this energetic structure ceases to exist once a person dies.

In its role as the life force, Ki is always present and active within the body. Moreover, Ki affects and even controls a person's entire life structure. To the Eastern mind, the unobstructed, balanced flow of Ki along the meridians is both the cause and the effect of good health. Eastern medicine including the disciplines of acupuncture and Shiatsu is dedicated to maintaining the balanced flow of Ki throughout the body, and to reestablishing that balance whenever it is thrown askew.

## THE STRUCTURE OF MERIDIANS

All bodily processes are associated with various major functions, each of which is in turn associated with one or more meridians. Consequently, each meridian has been assigned the name of an organ. (Because the relationship of a meridian to an organ is metaphorical rather than anatomical, many Westerners become confused when they find, for example, that the lung meridian lies along the arm, or that the liver meridian lies along the leg. The name assigned to a meridian refers not to the meridian's external location on the body but to the functional influence of the meridian within the body.) Table 22–1 contains a list of some of the major functions and the meridians with which they are associated.

These general functions illustrate the range of roles Ki plays in the human body and how the meridians work symbolically through the physiologic system. The theory of the life cycle of the meridians explains the sequence and the purpose of the various processes for maintaining life.

**TABLE 22–1.  FUNCTIONS ASSOCIATED WITH MAJOR MERIDIANS**

| Function | Meridians |
| --- | --- |
| Intake of Ki | Lung |
| Process of elimination | Large Intestine |
| Intake of food | Stomach |
| Digestion | Spleen |
| Interpretation of the emotional environment | Heart |
| Assimilation | Small Intestine |
| Purification | Bladder |
| Impetus to move | Kidney |
| Circulation | Heart Constrictor |
| Protection | Triple Heater |
| Storage, distribution, | Liver |
| and detoxification of Ki | Gall Bladder |

*Modified from S. Masunaga & W. Ohashi. (1977). Zen Shiatsu. Tokyo: Japan Publications, pp. 42–47.*

The cycle begins with the lung and large intestine meridians. As a pair, these meridians govern the intake of Ki and elimination. The action of inhaling the Ki from the outside world and bringing it into the body is represented by the respiratory system. The action of exhaling the extraneous Ki is represented by the eliminative system. On a symbolic level, the breath begins life by differentiating between the Ki from the outside world and the Ki within the human form. An example of this is the birth of a child. A child is not acknowledged as being alive until it takes its first breath. Once the child continues to breathe, its existence as a human being is established. The Ki from the outside world is separated from human Ki by the existence of a border, represented by the skin. The skin acts in two ways: (1) it absorbs Ki from the outside; and (2) it excretes waste material from the inside of the body via the pores. If both activities are in balance, the human form remains an entity.

Once this is established, two requirements are necessary for survival: (1) nourishment from an outside source; and (2) emotional stimuli to satisfy the spirit.

## Outside Nourishment

The primary external source of nourishment is food. Therefore, the intake of food and its breakdown for human consumption as represented in the process of digestion is an important function that is necessary in order to replenish expended Ki. The stomach and spleen meridians initiate these functions via the actual stomach, esophagus, and duodenum as well as via the digestive enzymes necessary for the breakdown of food.

## Emotional Stimuli

The second requirement is nourishment of the psyche by giving meaning to all human actions. The heart and small intestine meridians act as the interpreter and assimilator of stimuli that affect the emotions and feelings. A person's interaction with others is dependent on these functions; if a person cannot understand and absorb stimuli from the environment, life has no meaning beyond pure existence, and the reason for relationships and experiences ceases to exist. Of all the meridians, the heart and small intestine are most associated with the spiritual aspect of Ki, primarily compassion. They are the connecting links between the physical and heavenly bodies (i.e., our relation to the universe). On a physiologic level, the qualities of the heart are symbolized by the color red in our blood. Therefore, the heart and small intestine meridians are said to influence the quality of the blood.

These three pairs of meridians all deal with extracting Ki from the environment. When that function is completed, the Ki is then processed internally so it can be utilized. The first step is to filter out the impurities in the Ki taken in from the outside world and move it to the meridians that circulate it throughout the body. The bladder and kidney meridians govern the purification and movement process via urination, the autonomic nervous system, and the endocrine gland system.

When the Ki is refined, it is sent to the central distributors for circulation and protection. The heart constrictor and triple heater meridians are the central distributors that make Ki available to all parts of the body regardless of whether the body is active or inactive. In order for circulation to occur, a specific temperature must be maintained. The heart constrictor and triple heater meridians carry out these functions via the vascular system, the lymphatic system, and the metabolic processes that regulate body temperature.

When the Ki is available for use, the liver and gall bladder meridians control how the Ki is distributed to accomplish a specific action. For example, in the action of walking, more Ki would be channeled into the moving leg than other parts of the body that are still. However, not all the Ki is distributed and used. Much of it is stored for future use so that it does not have to be constantly replenished. The quality of Ki is constantly maintained through the process of detoxification. This function of allocating Ki for specific actions over a period of time parallels the birth and growth cycle whereby specific actions at different time periods contribute to a pattern of development. This function is represented on the physiologic level in the reproductive system. The liver and gall bladder meridians thus govern the reproductive system. Since life is a process, this cycle is ongoing until life ends.

The meaning of these functions can be interpreted on a variety of different levels including the physical, the emotional, the intellectual, and the spiritual. For example, an imbalance exhibited in the small intestine meridian indicates that the process of assimilation may not be working properly. On the physical plane, this imbalance may indicate faulty absorption of nutrients from the food in the intestines. This imbalance may express itself through physical symptoms such as acne, flatulence, migraine headaches, and intestinal problems. If the remedy addresses the problem of assimilation, the physical symptoms will automatically subside.

On an emotional plane, an assimilation problem might occur if there is an overload of emotional stimuli coming from the environment. Having to process and cope with the reactions to such stimuli disrupts the assimilation mechanism that normally adds meaning to our emotional environment. In cases such as trauma when the person cannot cope with the amount of stimuli derived from the experience, the body halts the assimilation process by going into a state of shock. This imbalance might manifest itself in symptoms such as hypersensitivity, the inability to cope with emotional situations, or the inability to recall traumatic experiences (in cases of shock).

On an intellectual plane, a small intestine meridian imbalance may indicate an inability to fully understand abstract concepts and an inability to follow through on details. Symptoms could include excessive worrying, anxiety, or too much concentration on unimportant details.

On a spiritual plane, an assimilation problem may exhibit itself by a person's being overwhelmed with emotion during religious experiences or by a lack of compassion due to an inability to react emotionally.

We can see from this analysis that a variety of symptoms can manifest themselves from one single cause—in this case, poor assimilation. If the imbalance in a particular meridian is rectified, it will have positive repercussions on all of the different planes.

## HOMEOSTASIS

*Homeostasis* is a modern scientific term that happens to describe quite suitably the flow of Ki within and among the meridians. The idea behind homeostasis is that dynamic systems (in this case the human body) naturally seek and maintain a condition of overall balance. Whenever an external force is applied to the system, at least one change must occur in the system in order to establish a new condition of balance.

With regard to the balance of Ki, external forces resulting from physical, mental, and spiritual stresses produce internal obstructions that are released at points along the meridians, termed *tsubos*. The character of these obstructions depends not only on the meridian or meridians affected but also on the quality and quantity of the Ki involved in the imbalance. The study of the quality and quantity of Ki and how it influences homeostasis in the body involves the concepts of vibration quality and of Kyo-Jitsu.

### Vibration Quality

Ki can be thought of as a form of vibration that ranges in frequency from low to high. Ki with a low vibrational quality seems heavy and slow, whereas Ki with a high vibrational quality seems light and fast. These qualities are additionally influenced by the quantity of Ki present, which can be either deficient or excessive. The most common sensations of vibration felt are temperature differences, i.e., high vibration is sensed in heat and low vibration is sensed in the feeling of coldness. However, these are not the only barometers for measuring the quality of vibration. Trained Shiatsu practitioners spend years developing sensitivity to the flow of Ki within the body and are able to feel subtle vibrational qualities of energy imbalances associated with illness, disease, and pain.

### Kyo-Jitsu[4]

The terms kyo and jitsu refer to the quantity as well as quality of Ki. *Kyo* is defined as an area of deficient and weak Ki, whereas *jitsu* is defined as an area of excessively strong Ki. Imbalances generally stem from an absence of Ki (kyo) because this absence retards a meridian's function. When this occurs, the life process is threatened and the remainder of the network becomes distorted as energy is redistributed in order to compensate for the weak area that is malfunctioning. As a consequence of this dynamic redistribution of energy, areas of excess Ki (jitsu) appear and are necessary to sustain the distorted state. This condition persists as long as the malfunction-

---

[4]Shizuto Masunaga & Wataru Ohashi. (1977). *Zen Shiatsu*. Tokyo: Japan Publications, p. 38.

ing area remains weak. Once the weakness is alleviated, the meridian initially affected regains its normal function, the remainder of the body is able to disperse the areas of jitsu, and the normal pattern of energy flow becomes reestablished.

## TYPES OF SHIATSU

Presently, there are three major types of Shiatsu being practiced, each of which approaches the goal of balancing energy flow differently: Shiatsu massage, acupressure, and *Zen* Shiatsu.

As explained earlier, Shiatsu massage is based largely on Anma techniques and views the body purely from an anatomical or physiologic perspective. In conjunction with the use of massage techniques and manipulations, hard pressure is applied to the body at certain points to elicit the relief of specific symptoms. The most widely known form of Shiatsu massage is the Namikoshi method.[5]

Acupressure is similar to Shiatsu massage, the difference being that acupressure incorporates the same theory of meridians and tsubos used by acupuncture. Acupressure is advocated in books by Katsusuke Serizawa,[6] and is discussed in Chapter 20 of this book.

Perhaps the most recent style of Shiatsu to gain recognition, Zen Shiatsu recognizes a broader set of meridians and tsubos than does acupuncture (Fig. 22–1). The level of pressure applied to the tsubos and meridians is significantly lighter than that in other types of Shiatsu. Also, unlike Shiatsu massage and acupressure, Zen Shiatsu incorporates the diagnostic theory of kyo-jitsu. This style of Shiatsu was developed by the late Shizuto Masunaga, founder and director of the Iokai Shiatsu Center in Japan. Because this style of Shiatsu is unique, its basic concepts will be discussed in detail.[7] (Hereafter, the term *Shiatsu* will be used to mean Zen Shiatsu.)

## THE ROLE OF THE SHIATSU PRACTITIONER

The Shiatsu practitioner has three primary goals: diagnosis (to identify the nature and extent of energy imbalances in a patient), treatment (to penetrate meridians in such a way as to alleviate the imbalances that exist), and maintenance (to apply manual pressure in such a way as to sustain and strengthen the existing energy balance).

---

[5]Tokujiro Namikoshi. (1969). *Shiatsu*. San Francisco: Japan Publications; and Toru Namikoshi. (1981). *The complete book of Shiatsu therapy*. Tokyo: Japan Publications. For a complete discussion of the Namikoshi method, read these texts.
[6]Katsusuke Serizawa. (1976). *Tsubo*. Tokyo: Japan Publications; and (1984). *Effective tsubo therapy*. Tokyo: Japan Publications. For a complete discussion of acupressure, read these texts.
[7]Shizuto Masunaga & Wataru Ohashi. (1977). *Zen Shiatsu*. Tokyo: Japan Publications. For a complete discussion of Zen Shiatsu, read this text.

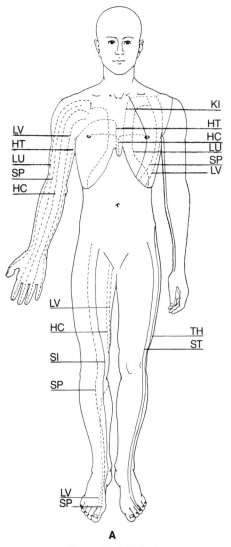
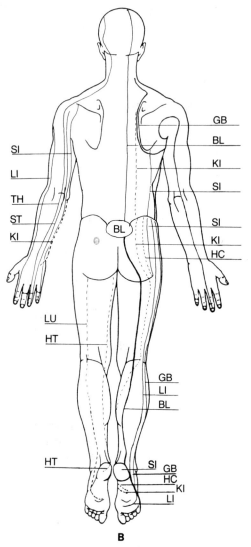

A

B

**Figure 22–1A&B.** Meridians used in Zen Shiatsu. Meridians pool in the abdominal area, shown in Figure 22–2, where they are touched for diagnostic purposes only. Meridians shown on one side of the body for schematic simplicity are the same on both sides. Key: LU-Lung; LI-Large Intestine; ST-Stomach; SP-Spleen; HT-Heart; SI-Small Intestine; BL-Bladder; KI-Kidney; HC-Heart Constrictor (Pericardium); TH-Triple Heater; LV-Liver; and GB-Gall Bladder. *(For a more detailed illustration of Masunaga's meridians, see Masunaga, S. & Ohashi, W. (1977).* Zen Shiatsu, *Tokyo: Japan Publications, p. 22.)*

## DIAGNOSIS

The underlying purpose of diagnosis in Shiatsu is to identify the cause and effect relationship between a kyo meridian and a jitsu meridian, with the goal of altering the cause of the condition so that the effect will take care of itself. (In any cause-and-effect relationship, the effect will persist until the cause is dealt with. For instance, a person lacking adequate food will feel continuously hungry. Once he or she eats, however, the hunger disappears.) Specifically, a jitsu condition (the effect) disperses automatically once the weak kyo condition (the cause) is altered. Because diagnostic areas for each of the 12 meridians are located in the abdomen (Fig. 22–2), the primary means of evaluating the state of a person's energy is to palpate the abdominal area. The intent is to use findings of kyo and jitsu areas to identify those meridians in which energy levels and flow are out of balance. (Additional sites on the back can be used for visual diagnosis. When there is

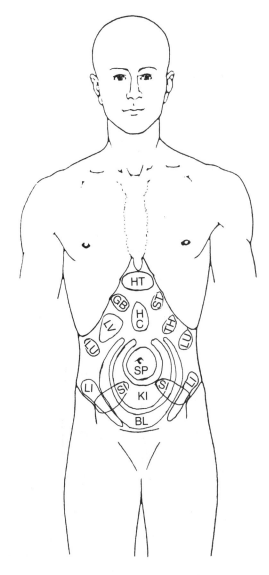

**Figure 22-2.** Diagnostic areas in the abdomen for the 12 meridians.

an imbalance in a meridian, the area where it pools in the back may appear distorted or out of proportion to the whole [Fig. 22–3].)

Skill in diagnosis is a function of the practitioner's ability to sense kyo and jitsu relationships within the abdomen. Once those relationships have been correctly identified, a talented practitioner can usually draw meaningful conclusions as to how and why the imbalance developed. Typically, a Shiatsu session begins with palpation of the patient's abdomen; pressure is then applied to tsubos along the kyo and jitsu meridians; finally, the abdomen is once again palpated. If the practitioner has been effective, the final palpation will indicate that both the kyo and jitsu conditions have been altered and even alleviated entirely.

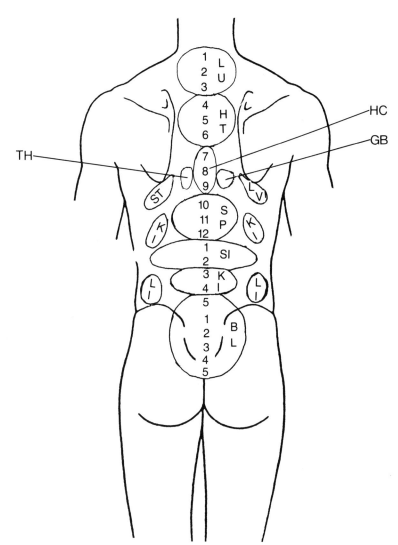

**Figure 22-3.** Diagnostic areas in the back for the 12 meridians.

## SHIATSU TECHNIQUES

Four primary principles govern Shiatsu techniques:

1. The giver maintains the attitude of an observer.
2. Penetration is perpendicular to the surface of the meridian being treated.
3. Body weight rather than strength is used to allow the hand to penetrate into the meridian that is being worked on.
4. Pressure is applied rhythmically.

### The Practitioner as Observer

In order to tap into the body's natural source of healing energy so that it can remedy an imbalance, the Shiatsu practitioner must become attuned to the internal dynamics of the Ki structure of the body by the simple device of observation. Maintaining a relaxed hand and an attitude devoid of any intention to interfere with the receiver's Ki, the practitioner ensures that the focus remains on using the receiver's own energy as the source of healing. The practitioner acts as a catalyst for the healing process.

### Perpendicular Penetration

The purpose of Shiatsu is to effect changes in the flow of energy in a meridian by manipulating the energy vortices called tsubos. However, contacting the flow of Ki in a meridian is analagous to pouring water into a vase. (The word *tsubo* in Japanese means *vase*. The metaphor is of a vessel with a narrow neck.) Unless water is poured into the vase from directly overhead, much will be lost. Similarly, in Shiatsu, penetration into the tsubo must occur at a 90-degree angle to the tsubo in order to have the optimum impact on the flow of Ki within the meridian. At any other angle, the effects will remain on the surface and will not penetrate deeply enough to influence the meridian.

Shiatsu techniques that employ perpendicular penetration produce significant changes in the meridian structure that go beyond superficial stimulation.

### Body Weight Versus Muscle Strength

The type of pressure applied directly affects the nature of the impact a Shiatsu session has on the receiver. To apply hard pressure to a meridian, the practitioner would have to tense the upper-body muscles forcefully; to endure such hard pressure, the receiver would have to remain totally passive and would be unable to participate at all in the healing process. Since tension decreases a practitioner's sensitivity, no communication bond between giver and receiver could be established. The practitioner would dominate the process, and the receiver would remain a passive recipient. Techniques that utilize hard pressure require more upper-body strength than do more gentle techniques, and they can produce physical problems in the shoulders and arms of the giver.

In contrast, when penetration of tsubos is achieved through the use of body weight, the practitioner's hand and upper body remain relaxed rather than tense. Pressure is applied by transferring the body's weight into the hand. The receiver senses this type of pressure as firm but gentle, with the result that a communication line of energy is established between giver and receiver. This relaxed form of penetration draws the receiver's own energy into the area being touched. The receiver participates by using that energy to rectify the imbalance in the meridian. The communication bond enables the practitioner to detect changes as they take place in the meridian and thereby monitor the receiver's response and progress. Because giver and receiver are providing each other feedback, this type of Shiatsu is beneficial to both.

## Rhythm

The receiver's response to Shiatsu is contingent on the quality of the pressure being used on the meridians and tsubos. The intervals at which pressure is felt constitute the rhythmic pattern of the technique. The response to rhythm can be seen in a person's response to music. If a piece of music has a slow rhythm, the common reaction to it is one of relaxation or of feeling soothed. A slow rhythm also allows the listener to focus on the composition of the music and how each note is played in relation to the others. If the rhythm is fast, the listener reacts excitedly, responding by moving the body or dancing. Instead of tuning in to the notes being played, the person is carried away with the active response to the beat.

The rhythms of Shiatsu technique elicit similar responses. A slow rhythm is produced when perpendicular pressure is held on a tsubo for a short length of time (usually the time needed to create a vibrational change in the area being touched). This is the principal technique used when working along the kyo meridian because it brings the cause of the imbalance to the attention of the receiver. This results in more permanent changes in the energy pattern. When the pressure is held, it allows the receiver's energy to tune in to the area of weakness and remedy it. At the same time, the slow rhythm relaxes and soothes, making it easier for the receiver to participate in the healing process.

A fast rhythm, on the other hand, causes the Ki in the tsubo being touched to disperse. Fast-moving, perpendicular pressure produces a rapid rhythm that distracts the receiver's attention from the cause of an imbalance. Because of this, sole use of this type of pressure throughout an entire Shiatsu session produces very temporary results. This technique is used primarily on the jitsu meridian to assist in the redistribution of excess Ki in an area that is exceptionally obstructed, as in cases of injury.

If these four primary guidelines are adhered to, Shiatsu becomes a highly effective method for correcting Ki imbalances quickly with the least amount of effort exerted by the giver. When this is accomplished, the healing power of both the giver and receiver are strengthened.

## BENEFITS OF SHIATSU

In Oriental medicine, a therapeutic approach was considered valid if it produced consistently positive results over a long period of time with little or no ill effect. This contrasts with Western medicine, in which the focus is on fast relief of the present symptoms in the shortest period of time, often without regard for the long-range effects. Although Western science still does not recognize the existence of the meridian structure of the body, there is no doubt that the practical application of the basic principles of Shiatsu work.

## SUMMARY

Humankind may have changed through the years, but the relationship of the human species to natural law has remained the same. Shiatsu is based on that law, and its tool, the hand, is imbued with the sensitive qualities necessary to evaluate the impact those laws are having on an individual. Just as the ancient system of meridians and tsubos is as effective today as it was thousands of years ago, Shiatsu continues to unify body, mind, and spirit and contribute to a life lived to its highest potential through healthful and fulfilling experiences.

# 23

# Polarity Therapy

Beverly Kitts, R.P.T.

Polarity therapy is an alternative holistic health care system involving exercises, nutrition, and love, as well as a system of gentle bodywork techniques. Unlike other forms of massage, Polarity involves simple touching rather than stroking. The therapist always has both hands on the client's body, either merely resting them in specific places, rocking the body, or rhythmically pressing in at various depths. These touches are designed to release obstructions to the free flow of energy through the body, so that the person is supported in returning to health.

## HISTORY

Polarity therapy was developed in the middle 1900s by Randolph Stone, chiropractor, naturopath, and osteopathic physician. Stone was intrigued by the thought that there must be a basic principle underlying the effectiveness of diet change, manipulations, exercise, and other natural cures. Why did the same health problem respond positively to diet change in one person, spinal manipulation in another, and exercise in another? Why did some people seem predisposed to illness, whereas others seemed to have an innate vitality?

The search for this underlying principle led Stone to study Chinese acupuncture and herbal medicine, the Hermetic Cabalistic systems of the Middle East, and the ancient Ayurvedic medicine of India. In each of these traditions, he found two complementary elements—the belief in a subtle form of life energy that permeates the body and gives it health, and the understanding that disease is a result of obstruction to that flow of energy. Stone theorized that all natural healing techniques are effective because they support the individual's innate capacity for health by stimulating the free and balanced flow of life energy. He combined his Western skills with techniques from all the Eastern traditions he had studied, and explored them from the unique vantage point of their effect on the subtle life energy.

Stone then spent many years practicing methods for freeing energy flow and studying meditation in India. Indian philosophical framework permeates his writings on Polarity. The life energy is described in terms of longitudinal, horizontal, and diagonal lines of force, *chakras* (energy centers in the body), and the five elements (earth, water, fire, air, and ether). Foods, hands-on work, and exercises are discussed according to their effect on the balancing of these elements. This rather esoteric aspect of Polarity, along with the incorporation of chiropractic and osteopathic techniques, makes his writings difficult for the average reader.

After Stone's retirement in 1973, Pierre Pannetier began to spread the practice of Polarity across the United States through seminars. Pannetier did much to systematize the series of physical mobilizations and make the more esoteric nature of Stone's work accessible to the lay practitioner.

However, the very eclectic nature of Stone's teaching makes it difficult to actually define Polarity. In its truest sense, *Polarity* includes *anything* that promotes life. Through the years, different practitioners have tended to incorporate whatever supplemental skills they might have, and rightly so, in order to best support the health of the client. Various schools of Polarity that have sprung up are very different from each other in style of hands-on work, amount of pressure used, emphasis on esoterica, and supplemental skills such as training in Gestalt therapy.

Many Polarity therapists emphasize the esoteric aspect of the tradition, and may use this framework to explain or develop their sessions, "I am working with your fire current, as an imbalance in it is undermining the health of your sinuses." However, acceptance of the esoteric aspects is not at all essential to the practice of Polarity. Pannetier often advised his students to forget their intellects, including all thoughts based on Ayurveda. He would instruct them to sense the obstructions with their hands and work intuitively in that present moment of touching, using Stone's manipulations as springboards and developing new ones as needed. There is a vast wealth of powerful and effective techniques in the system of Polarity, and this attention to intuition is in no way meant to downplay or degrade the value of learning technique. It is simply that the practitioner must learn to go beyond the intellect's limitations into the direct experience of working with the subtle energies.

Studying Polarity is similar to studying music—many "scales" are practiced, new "melodies" and "styles" are learned in order to stretch the student's capacity and stimulate creativity. Theory can be a valuable aid, but is not essential. The desired end result is to play from one's heart in a responsive manner that is open to the needs of the present moment.

## PHYSIOLOGY OF HANDS-ON WORK

To date, Western science has expressed little interest in researching this so-called "life energy." Although we have yet to reach scientific understanding of what happens during Polarity therapy, something does happen. There are subjective as well as objective indications that some principle not yet recognized by Western medicine is involved.

- Subjectively, health is often equated with being full of energy, whereas the first sign of impending illness is often its absence.
- Subjectively, the therapist feels a definite tingling in his or her hands when doing the various mobilizations. The degree and pattern of this tingling vary with the state of health of the area being worked, and they change as the area is treated.
- Subjectively, the patient and therapist often note simultaneous changes in their sense of energy. The receiver feels freer, lighter, more relaxed; the therapist notes a balancing and strengthening of the tingling in his or her hands, and a sense of an overall increase in energy.

The Polarity therapist views these changes as a response to unblocking the life energy by affecting muscular relaxation, structural change, and balancing the autonomic nervous system. Western medicine would probably say that the tingling is simply vasodilation in the hands; the talk of energy is pseudoscience; the positive health gains are a result of the placebo effect.

Yet, Western science would also have to note that there are objective changes taking place. After just a few minutes of Polarity therapy, signs of deep relaxation appear. Often, cheeks flush, blood pressure drops, salivation increases, the heart rate slows, the eyes may tear, and the stomach and intestines may grumble with the increase in peristalsis. These are objective signs of a relaxation response from the parasympathetic nervous system. It is interesting to note that this response to Polarity is often far more dramatic than the response to Swedish massage.

Closer examination reveals clear physiologic rationales for the effectiveness of many of the specific techniques. Many can be seen as stimulation to nerve centers. For example, one commonly given technique involves very light oscillating pressure over the pressure-sensitive Baro receptors in the carotid arteries along the sides of the neck. It is probable that, although the pressure is so slight as to cause no interference with the blood supply to the brain, it is sufficient to activate the neurologic reflex signal that slows the heart rate and lowers blood pressure. This same reflex is usually triggered by stretching of the Baro receptors from within when the blood pressure going to the brain is too high.

Polarity often utilizes rocking motions of the limbs and trunk. These vary from small, gentle oscillations to large, vigorous oscillations that move the entire body. This rocking commonly induces relaxation, lowers muscle tone, reduces pain, and encourages an increase in the active range of motion afterward. Western medicine is just beginning to be aware of the tremendous benefits of this pain-free way of stimulating the joint mechanoreceptors, the nerve endings that receive messages about movements in the joints. It appears that when these receptors are gently stimulated, a reflex response will lower muscle tone, increase circulation, and stimulate endorphin release, which results in a decrease in pain sensation.

In addition, it appears that the alternating rhythmic manner with which the two hands are used and the style of touch often induce a light hypnotic trance. Patients frequently report experiencing an unusual mind state in which they feel as though every part of their body and mind were relaxed and even asleep, except for their simple awareness of sensory stimuli. This state of deepened relaxation lays the foundation for health and well-being by returning the body and mind to a state of balanced homeostasis. Even if only temporary, the moments of peace provided by a Polarity session are a much needed experience in this stressful culture. In addition, this state of quiet awareness allows people to see their problems from a broader perspective, often seeing solutions that had previously been buried by the noisiness of the conscious mind. Hidden feelings may surface, making Polarity therapy an excellent adjunct to psychotherapeutic work. Thus, although Western science does not view energy as a structurally existing entity, it would seem apparent that, functionally, the human body responds to the Polarity touch in a manner that supports health of the body and mind.

It is interesting to note how many of the techniques are as easily set within the framework of modern medicine as they are within Ayurvedic philosophy. It is as though the basic principle Stone sought transcends all ideas, ancient or modern, and is instead embodied in the actual experience of the hands-on work, rather than in the particular theories used to explain it. Energy is simply an abstracted metaphor—one way of looking at the results obtained through Polarity. Neurologic reflex is another abstracted metaphor—a way of explaining a mechanism we cannot see, except in its effects.

## PRINCIPLES OF POLARITY THERAPY

### Energy

Working with energy is a concept foreign to most Westerners. And yet it is not as difficult or unusual as we might expect. In this culture, not much time or value is placed on subtle awareness of changes in the hands. A simple experiment can show how these sensations can be picked up and amplified. Rub the palms of your hands together, waking the nerve endings and bringing your awareness to your palms. Then hold them about 6 in apart; relax, and center your awareness, amplifying incoming sensory input by focusing. Experiment with moving your hands closer and farther apart to see if and how the feeling changes. Then move the hands so that the palms are no longer facing, and be aware of how they feel.

Many people find that when the palms are facing each other, there is a tingling sensation of relatedness, as though the hands were "plugging into" each other. Try the same sequence with your eyes closed; from the sensation or its absence you may know whether or not your palms are directly opposite each other.

## Love

The foremost principle espoused in Polarity therapy is the importance of working with love. Pannetier used to say that love was the most vital element of the whole session. He would say, "If you don't know what to do, just put your hands on the person and love them."

What is this love? Obviously it is not sloppy sentimentality, or an overbearing affection. Beyond that, it is difficult to put into words. Trying to act in a loving manner, or matching an idea of what we think Pannetier is talking about, misses again. To really love is a matter quite different from holding an idea about love. This love of which he spoke has no objective, not even that of healing the patient, or helping someone. It is a caring so powerful that it carries with it no agenda, no end result that must be obtained. The therapist does his or her work simply, always responding to the felt need, and yet without attachment to healing. This love is serving life. The therapist who "cares enough not to care," as Dylan Thomas once said, "can truly let go and trust in the universe." The seeds of this relaxation are then watered in the patient's own being. This fosters an extremely deep state of relaxation and trust. It is in this relaxed state that healing occurs, if it is meant to be.

Once the practitioner has begun to understand this principle, the rich wealth of Polarity techniques can be explored, but always with the understanding that it is not the particular technique that heals. This attitude of surrender and openness, this simple "getting out of the way" of the body's inherent tendency to homeostasis allows healing on many levels. Muscles relax, digestion improves, circulation increases in areas where it is needed, hormone levels normalize, endorphins increase, breathing deepens, and so on.

A good place to begin exploring this quality of love is a simple "front-to-back" Polarity technique. You will need a partner for this exercise.

Instruct your partner to sit on a stool or sideways in a chair so that the chest and thoracic area (upper back) are both easily accessible. Stand at the person's left side, and slowly and gently place your left palm over the person's heart and your right palm over the upper back between the shoulder-blades. Move your hands slowly around until you feel a sensation of the palms "plugging into each other," as though they were connected by a flow of energy (Fig. 23–1).

Simply hold your hands in place. Check your own posture to see that it

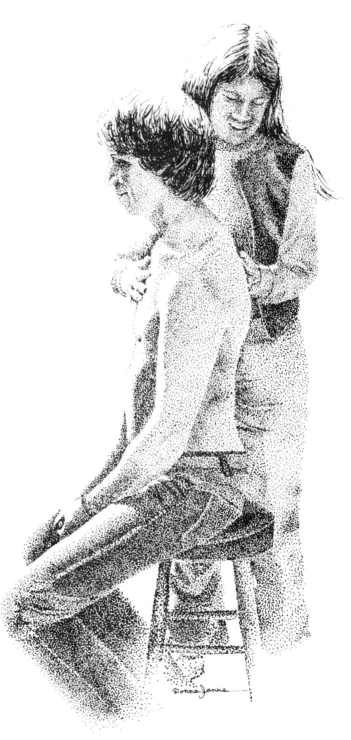

**Figure 23-1.** Feeling palms "plugging into each other."

is relaxed and that your breathing is natural and uncontrolled. After a bit, your palms may begin to tingle more or less strongly, or feel unusually warm. Some practitioners do not experience these signs, but feel an inner sense of rightness, an increasing sense of peace and completion. The experience is different for everyone. The patient may sigh, visibly relax, and show a change in his or her breathing pattern. You may feel a change in your hands, or in your mind state, at about the same time. After a few minutes, very slowly withdraw your hands.

Many therapists find that their discursive intellects are quite loud during this exercise, and that they are unable to tune into their hands or their subtle feelings. They are so busy watching for results or criticizing their own efforts that awareness of subtle changes in their hands is impossible. It takes practice and a continual "letting go" on the part of the therapist.

## Working the Obstructions

Another principle in Polarity is that the obstructions must be released for optimal results. An obstruction is an area of the body where there seems to be a stagnation or a holding pattern that somehow interferes with a free flow of energy. In simple terms, for example, a person who is experiencing chronic anxiety may have abdominal tension, disturbed peristalsis, and nausea. Their posture may be somewhat caved in, as though they were trying to protect themselves from imminent danger. If you were to look at such a person, you might imagine that any lines of energy trying to flow vertically through that person might be really disturbed in the abdominal–diaphragmatic area. The Polarity therapist would respond to these obstructed areas with techniques that would tend to release tension and encourage a free flow of naturally organized and balanced energy.

An alert Polarity therapist will begin assessing patients visually as soon as they walk in the door. The therapist will be looking for areas that seem out of alignment, do not move with the rest of the body when the patient walks, seem held or protected, etc. Further clues are found from the patient's self-reports, and by touch, as the bodywork session begins. The following exercise is designed to introduce you to the principle of finding and locating obstructions.

Have your partner lie supine, facing upward. Slowly and gently place your right palm on his or her abdomen between the navel and the pubic bone. You may sense tension or the opposite—flaccidity—in the musculature. You can become alert to the breathing pattern. Does it seem restricted or unusually fast or slow? Does the breathing pattern change as you touch the person? You may sense irregularities in the skin temperature, or a tightness only in a certain area as though there were a pocket of gas under your hand. Make certain that your hand, wrist, elbow, and shoulder muscles are completely relaxed, and that your own breathing is calm. The touch should be light. If you are able to relax, you can increase the pressure slightly, first with the heel of the hand and then the fingers, alternating in wave-like motion (Fig. 23–2).

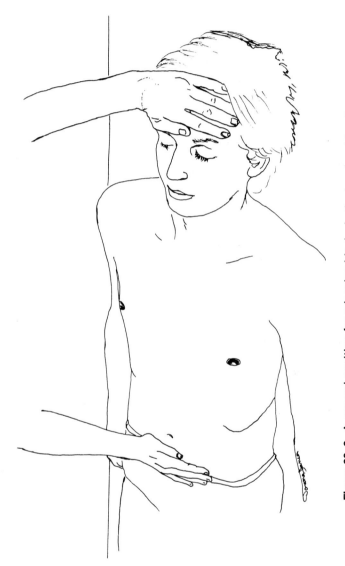

**Figure 23–2.** A general position for releasing blocks in the torso and head.

Leaving your right hand resting on the abdomen, place your left hand over your partner's forehead. With practice, you will be able to sense whether the head is held rigidly by the neck muscles, and whether the person is subtly moving toward or away from your hand. As you lightly touch, see if you can feel the sensation of your hands "plugging in" again. Feelings of warmth or tingling may begin in one or both hands. Gently rock the lower body a few minutes with the right hand, as though you were rocking a baby to sleep. The left hand should remain resting lightly on the forehead throughout, without rocking. As the sensation of connectedness or tingling increases, you may see signs of an increased energy flow. Your partner's face may show more color, muscles may relax, and the breathing may deepen and become more regular. You have helped melt areas of tension, or obstructions, in the areas under and between your two hands.

### Understanding

In the above exercise, it is also quite possible that your partner experienced the opposite of the relaxation response. At times, the muscular armoring has served an important function for the patient, helping him or her feel safer, for example. As these muscles release their tension, it is common for fear to arise. The person may be confused by this response, which can be of some magnitude. For this reason, many schools of Polarity include basic counselling skills. Pannetier used a commonsense approach emphasizing a caring attitude, acceptance, and trust that whatever happens is from the "clearing of blocks" and is for the best.

Polarity is a gentle art. The therapist invites the patient to enter a deeply relaxed state and invites muscles to relax. Nothing is ever forced. Pannetier would often say that no harm can come from Polarity so long as the touch is gentle enough not to override the patient's natural tendency to homeostasis. If the patient wishes to enter into and pass through the feeling of obstruction the therapist will continue to work with areas of holding, deepening the relaxation, allowing the energy flow between the hands to build and balance. If the patient wishes to pull away from the experience, reassurance can be given and alternate areas can be worked that are not threatening, perhaps building trust for work with the more tightly defended areas at a later time. It is often the case that as the patient lets go in other areas, highly charged areas may release without his or her conscious awareness.

Thus, Pannetier would say, it is vital for the therapist to have a proper understanding of personal responsibility. The patient is reaping the effects of past actions and present decisions. The therapist is not there to rescue the patient, but to plant seeds of letting go and trusting, to be an accepting friend. This attitude protects the therapist from taking on patients' ailments in a misguided attempt to heal.

### Nutrition and Exercise

Both nutrition and exercise take a prominent part in the therapeutic regimen. Commonsense stretching and toning, sometimes with the addition of sounds to stimulate the flow of energy, are suggested. Their selection is again based on the Ayurvedic concepts of freeing and balancing the life energy. The specific system of exercise is loosely derived from yoga, but it has become more eclectic as teachers have incorporated their own experiences and viewpoints. The one basic stretch is the youthful pose, or squatting posture. In this position, it is said, all the currents are stimulated and the cosmic forces are attracted for health and rejuvenation.

Dietary suggestions are primarily based on Ayurvedic theory, that is, on the energetic qualities of various foods. Patients are commonly led through a period of "cleansing," during which intake of certain foods is severely limited. Daily use of a *liver flush*, a drink made of garlic, olive oil, and lemon juice followed by specific herbal teas, is often recommended. A simple vegetarian diet is recommended for daily fare. It should be noted that the primary emphasis in Polarity is on eating with a relaxed mind state, rather than on the particulars of what is eaten. Just as in hands-on work, the subtle mental aspects of diet are far more important than the material aspects and serve as a foundation for digestion and assimilation of whatever is eaten.

The emphasis on eating nutritious foods while in a relaxed state of mind and on exercising in a balanced manner is certainly basic to a Western view of health. However, the particulars are controversial, and unless one is approaching Polarity in its entirety as an offshoot of Ayurvedic medicine, they are not essential to an appreciation of the hands-on technique. For this reason, the remaining section of this chapter will deal solely with the hands-on art of Polarity.

## BASIC POLARITY MOBILIZATIONS

Beginning students are taught a general session of 22 mobilizations that serve to stimulate and balance the entire body. The gentle holding, rocking, and probing techniques form a generally relaxing session and also aid the practitioner in locating areas that appear to be obstructed and in need of further work.

Some of these techniques are derived from osteopathy, craniopathy, or chiropracty of the 1930s and 1940s. Some were derived by Stone from observations made by psychics, or from his study of acupuncture or Egyption medicine. Some were derived from theories of harmonic resonance—that certain parts of the body will vibrate harmonically when other areas are worked. All in all, the techniques form a fascinating and rich array of moves that must be experienced and done in order to be appreciated.

Jules Older, a clinical psychologist, has an interesting comment in his book *Touching Is Healing.*

> As with psychotherapy, there are many schools of massage, each more or less convinced that its specialized technique or underlying rationale is more efficacious than the others. Their names tell much about their

origins: Swedish, Esalen, Shiatsu, Acupressure, Polarity, Applied Kinesiology, Rolfing. Some stroke, others press, still others prod and jab. But whatever the differences in origin, theory or technique, I believe that it is only the territory that they share that is of real importance. As with psychotherapy the belief system of the masseur is of little consequence compared to what actually goes on in the room with the client. . . . I have found that a person with beliefs about the meaning of massage as different from mine as Mars is from marzipan can still give me a most wonderful going-over while one whose beliefs I share entirely can dish out some pretty indifferent stuff. It's not what's in their heads that matters so much as what goes on where skin meets skin.[1]

What follows is an abbreviated version of the General Session of Polarity therapy. The ideal supplement to this introductory chapter would be to receive a Polarity session from a professional therapist, as it is very difficult to convey in writing what the experience of Polarity is like. Polarity is truly an art form, requiring much study and dedicated practice in order to master the rhythm and quality of touch that are so important to the effects. In addition, the hands-on work is only a small part of the therapy, which usually includes basic nutritional guidance, exercise, and support for emotional balancing.[2]

## Abbreviated General Session[3]

Position: Have the person lie on her back on the massage table, while you sit on a chair at her head.

1. The tenth cranial ("the cradle"). Overlap the last three fingers of your left hand on the last three fingers of your right hand, palms up, to form a cradle (Fig. 23–3). Rest your hands on the table, supporting the person's head in your palms.

   Your index fingers should extend along the grooves beside the sternocleidomastoid muscle (where the carotid artery and tenth cranial nerve travel. Rest your thumbs on your index fingers rather than over the patient's ears. Hold one to two min, or until the current is strongly felt (Fig. 23-4).

2. Neck stretch. Rest the patient's head on the palm of your right hand, so that your first or second finger and thumb can take a firm hold on the base of her skull. Your left hand rests lightly on her forehead with your left thumb on the anterior fontanel (the "soft spot" in an infant). With firm steady pressure from the right hand

---

[1]Copyrighted © by Jules Older. (1983). *Touching is healing*. New York: Stein & Day, p. 101. Reprinted with permission.

[2]Readers desiring further information about training are encouraged to contact the American Polarity Therapy Association, PO Box 19459, Seattle, Washington 98109.

[3]For purposes of simplicity, the patient will be referred to consistently as "her."

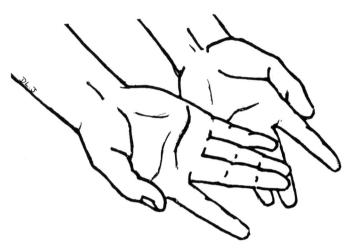

**Figure 23-3.** Hand position for "the cradle."

only, apply gentle traction toward you. As the patient exhales, slightly release; as she inhales, slightly increase the traction. This move is contraindicated if the patient is known to be hypermobile, or if there is any increase in pain in the arms, shoulders, neck, or head (Fig. 23–5).

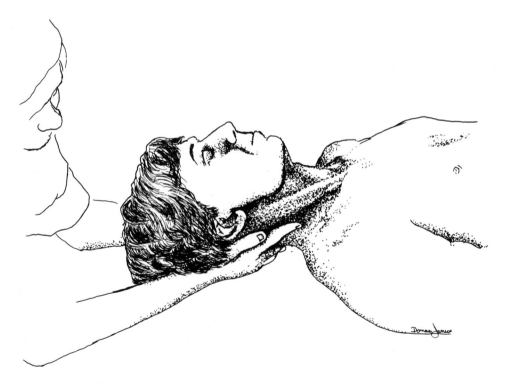

**Figure 23-4.** "The cradle."

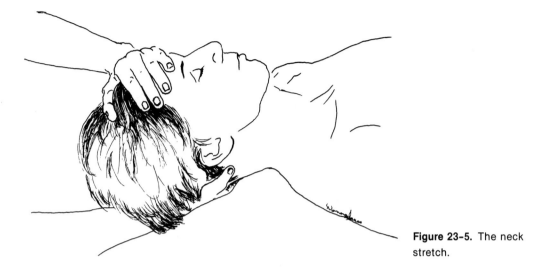

**Figure 23-5.** The neck stretch.

3. Tummy rock. Standing on the patient's right side, rest your left hand on her forehead, and your right hand on her abdomen half way between the navel and the pubic bone. Rock the abdomen gently, trying to tune into the person's natural "rocking rhythm." This mobilization was also described earlier, as a means of releasing blocks in the torso and head (Fig. 23–6).

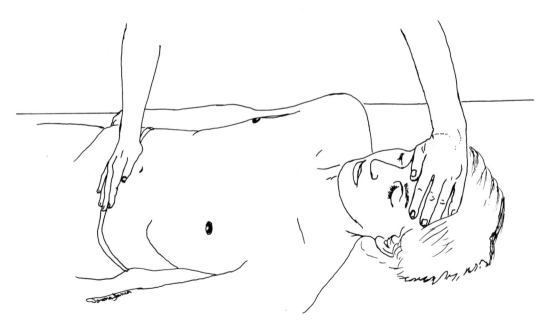

**Figure 23-6.** The tummy rock.

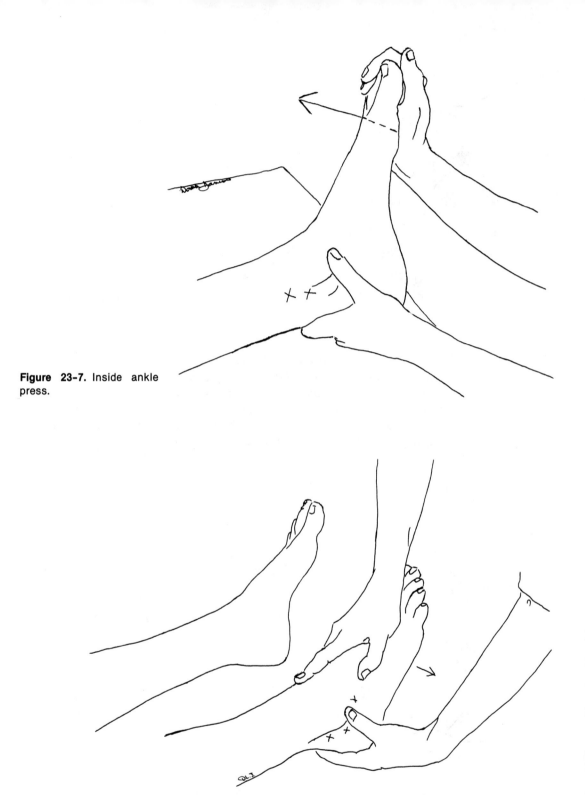

**Figure 23-7.** Inside ankle press.

**Figure 23-8.** Outside ankle press.

4. Leg pull. Grasp both feet behind the heels and gently pull legs straight towards you several inches off the ground. Check to see if one leg is shorter than the other, as there are specific treatments for the several causes of leg-length discrepancy. Rest the legs back on the table gently, and place your hands over the feet for a few moments before proceeding.

5. Inside ankle press. You can sit on a stool at your patient's feet if that is more comfortable for you than standing. Support the heel of her right foot with your left hand. With your right thumb, press gently in an arc under the inner ankle bone (medial malleolus). Pay special attention to any tender areas, applying rhythmic gentle compression until the points are pain free. Keeping your right hand in place, press on the ball of the foot with your left hand to flex the ankle forward (dorsiflexion). With practice, you will be able to alternate rhythmically between pressing an ankle point and flexing the ankle (Fig. 23–7).

6. Outside ankle press. Now, support the heel of her right foot with your left hand. (If the patient has a markedly externally rotated hip, you may need to lift the entire leg and rest it in your palm in a more neutral position in order to have the outside of the ankle accessible for work.) With your right thumb, find any tender areas along the area under the outside ankle bone (lateral malleolus). With your right hand, press the top of the foot downward (plantarflexion) giving a good stretch. Alternate rhythmically as described above (Fig. 23–8).

   Repeat moves 5 and 6 on the left foot, with hands reversed.

7. Pelvis and knee rock. Hold the feet again for a moment, and move up to the person's right side. Place your left hand on her lower right abdomen, just above the leg crease, with the fingers pointing down towards the feet. Place your right hand just above the knee. Very gently apply pressure with the right hand in a rhythmic fashion, gently rocking her leg. Continue for 10 to 30 seconds. Allow the leg to slow and then to be still. Continue holding for 30 seconds or so, again being aware of any sensations you feel. Carefully and slowly remove your hands (Fig. 23–9).

8. Arm–shoulder rotations. Hold the patient's right wrist as shown in Figure 23–10. Controlling movement from the wrist, gently rotate the shoulder in a small circle, alternately compressing and distracting the shoulder point. Do this about ten times toward you and ten times away from you.

9. Thumb web/forearm stimulation. Using the thumb and finger of your left hand, squeeze the webbing between her thumb and finger, concentrating on any tender areas. Press the pad of your right thumb into a point 1 in below the elbow crease and ½ in from the inside of her arm. Rhythmically alternate stimulation with each hand (Fig. 23–11).

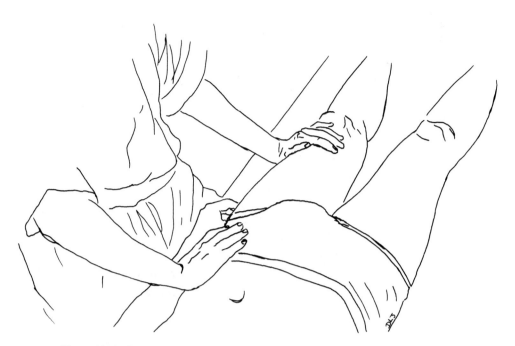

**Figure 23-9.** Pelvis and knee rock.

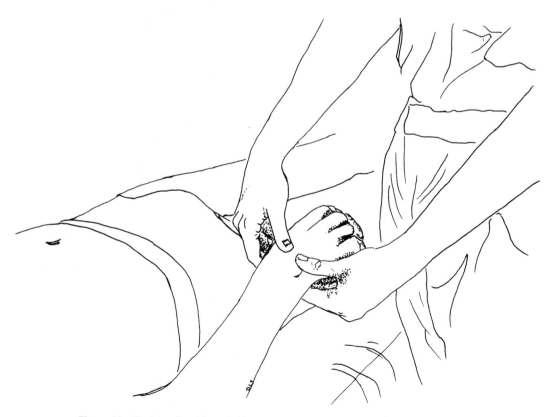

**Figure 23-10.** Arm-shoulder rotation.

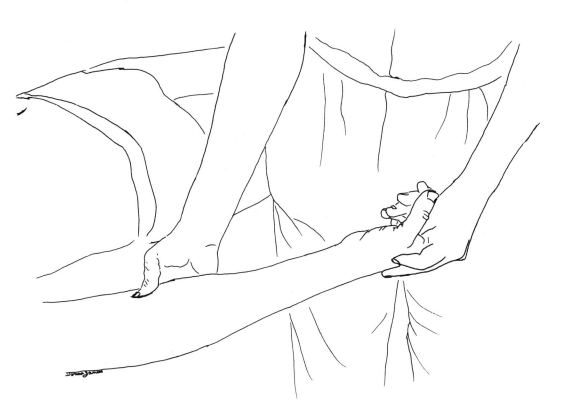

**Figure 23–11.** Thumb web/forearm stimulation.

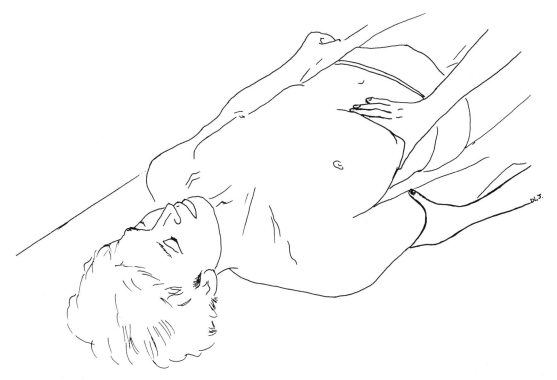

**Figure 23–12.** Elbow milk/abdomen rock.

213

10. Elbow milk/abdomen rock. Place your left hand under the patient's right elbow and lay your thumb across the elbow crease. Milk upwards with your thumb. Place your right hand lightly along the bottom edge of the rib cage, and gently rock the abdomen. Alternate milking and rocking, about 10 to 12 times each for roughly a minute (Fig. 23–12).

11. Pelvic rock. Place your right hand over the patient's left hip bone (anterior superior iliac spine). Place your left hand over her right shoulder. Stabilizing the shoulder girdle with your left hand, gently rock the trunk with the right. Gradually increase the rocking movement for 20 seconds, and then gradually decrease. Hold for a moment before moving on (Fig. 23–13).

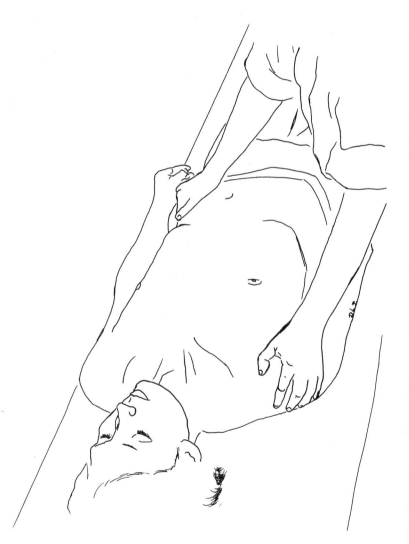

**Figure 23-13.** Pelvic rock.

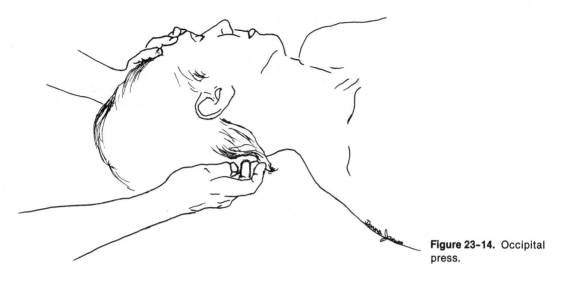

**Figure 23-14.** Occipital press.

Repeat moves 7 through 11 on the other side, with hands reversed.

12. Occipital press. Sitting at the patient's head, turn her head slightly to the left. Using the second finger of your right hand, give a rotational massage to the suboccipital muscles just under the base of the skull and to the right of the midline. Your left hand should be

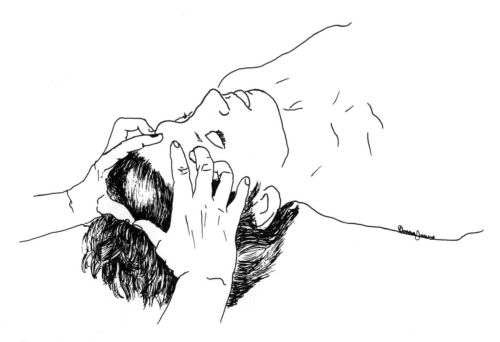

**Figure 23-15.** Cranial polarization.

supporting her head by resting lightly on the left side of her fore-head. Your index finger should rest gently on the spot known in India as the "third eye," the area between and just above the eyes. The hand on the back of the head should feel as though it were plugged into the palm of the hand on her forehead. Hold and feel for a sensation of tingling. When a steady gentle pulsation is felt in

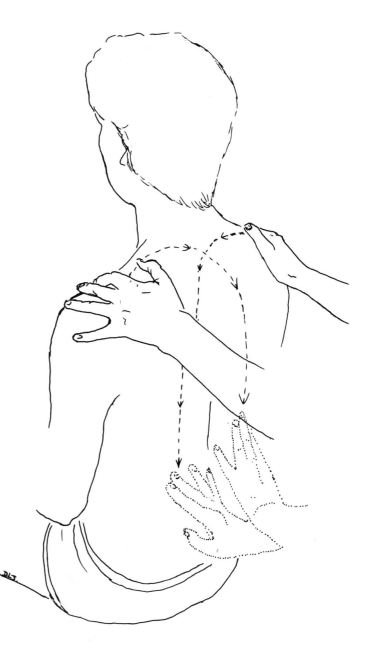

**Figure 23-16.** Brushing off the back.

the hands, or a minute or so has passed, turn the head to the other side and repeat, switching hands (Fig. 23–14).

13. Cranial polarization. Lightly place both thumbs on the anterior fontanel, with both index fingers touching on the "third eye" and the remaining fingers across the forehead. If your hands are large enough, rest your little fingers on the temperomandibular joints, with the other fingers evenly spaced on the forehead. It is important that you really relax your hands, arms, and shoulders as much as possible, and that your breathing is relaxed and your posture comfortable. Hold for about one min, or until a steady gentle pulsation is felt (Fig. 23–15).

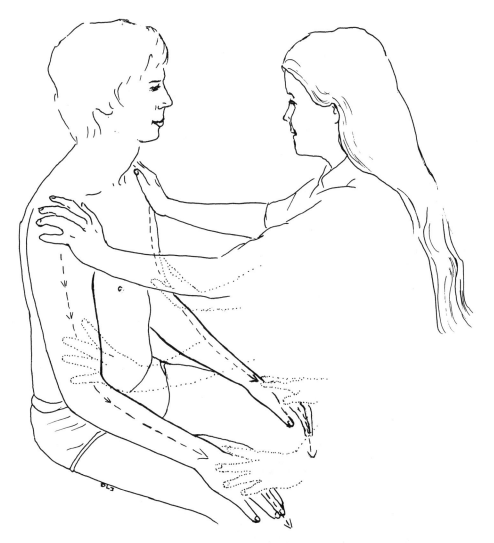

**Figure 23–17.** Brushing off the front.

14. Navel/third eye. Move to the patient's right side. Lightly place your left thumb pad between her eyebrows and your right thumb in her navel, with the thumbs pointing towards each other. Hold one min, and then lift hands very slowly, initiating movement from the thumbs, rather than the shoulders. Wait a few moments, and then in a quiet voice ask the patient to sit up with her legs off the side of the table. Standing behind her, place your hands on her shoulders. With a sweeping motion, brush your hands across the spine then down to the sacrum, and out to the crest of the hips. Repeat several times. Standing in front of her, place her hands on her knees. Place your hands on her shoulders, and in a sweeping manner, brush down her arms to the knees and down her legs. Repeat several times (Figs. 23–16 and 23–17).

If you decide to explore these techniques, remember the primary principle of love. If you get confused, let yourself laugh. If you find the rhythm difficult, remember to let your breathing relax, your shoulders down. If you are relaxed and accept yourself, your patient will benefit, regardless of your skill level. Do the best you can in a simple way, and be kind to yourself. Although you are not "the healer," you may find yourself being healed while giving Polarity. You may find that in the circle of love and self-acceptance your own obstructions begin to disappear and you are no longer sure who is "giving" Polarity to whom.

The unique gift of Polarity is its simplicity. Behind the techniques and esoterica is an opening and surrendering to life, and to being at home with our natural energies.

## References

Gordon, R. (1979). *Your healing hands: The Polarity experience.* Santa Cruz, CA: Unity Press.

Siedman, M. (1982). *Like a hollow flute: A guide to Polarity therapy.* Santa Cruz, CA: Elan Press.

Siegel, A. (1986). *Life energy: The power that heals.* Bridport, Dorset, England: Prism Press/Colin Spooner.

Stone, R. (For information about obtaining Dr Stone's book, (1986). *Polarity therapy: The complete collected works,* contact CRCS Publications, P.O. Box 20850, Reno, NV 89515.) His works include:
*Energy: The vital Polarity in the healing art.*
*Wireless anatomy of man and its function.*
*Supplement to wireless anatomy of man.*
*Polarity therapy in its triune function.*
*Vitality balance.*
*The mysterious sacrum.*
*Health building.*
*Easy stretching postures for vitality and beauty.*
*Appendix to the new energy concept.*
*Polarity therapy: Principles and practice.*

The author wishes to thank the artist Donna Janus for the excellent figures used to illustrate this chapter.

# — 24

# The Bindegewebsmassage System[1]

Both Eastern and Western medical philosophies assume that isolated pathologies do not exist anywhere in the human body. The entire organism functions as a balanced and coordinated unit if the body is healthy. Any disability that disrupts this harmony affects the autonomic and central nervous system as well as hormonal and humoral systems. In all cases the body must be considered as a physiological and psychological whole.

## PHYSIOLOGY OF BINDEGEWEBSMASSAGE

The most superficial layer of the tissues forming the body surface is the skin. It is the immediate link with the external environment. It contains the exteroceptors, i.e., specialized nerve endings that react to touch in various intensities and to changes in temperature such as heat and cold.

The deepest layer forming the body surface is that of the muscles. These also contain numerous nerve endings that can alter the tension in the tissue both reflexively and voluntarily. These nerve endings register alterations in the tension of the tissue by means of proprioceptors, i.e., specialized nerve

---

[1] The material presented in this chapter reflects the viewpoint of the Elisabeth Dicke School in Uberlingen, West Germany, where the author of this book studied. In addition to Dicke's *Meine Bindegewebsmassage* (Hippokrates-Verlag, Stuttgart, 1956), Marie Ebner's book, *Connective Tissue Massage* (Williams & Wilkins, Baltimore, 1962) was very helpful since it clarified many points that were difficult to understand in Dicke's text. However, the material in this chapter is Dicke's Bindegewebsmassage as the author learned it in Uberlingen, and it varies from Ebner's text in many ways.

endings sensitive to alterations in the length of the muscle fiber. Both these tissues relate to the somatic and the autonomic nervous systems. Therefore, vascular changes occur in both tissues.

The layer of tissue between skin and muscle consists of connective tissue, and this is the layer that is thought to be particularly important when applying Bindegewebsmassage.

It is considered that organic disturbances follow vascular channels over arterial reflexes. It is believed that these reactions are responsible for many pathologic disturbances that cannot be explained as reflex symptoms within the segmental distribution. The Bindegewebsmassage system of massage is based on the concept that these reactions are responsible for certain disabilities. This may explain the reason some cases claim removal of peripheral symptoms through massage of the connective tissue to the back. These segments do not correspond to the dermatome area in the periphery. (See Fig. 24–1 for the back areas that correspond to visceral pathologies described by MacKenzie.) This information is taken largely from German sources, but the beneficial effect of the treatment has been confirmed by the experiences of people of many nationalities.

At the beginning of a treatment program one should proceed cautiously to build up tolerance to these procedures. Begin with the basic strokes, the Grundaufbau. Then, if the patient tolerates it well, one can proceed to the thoracic and cervical segments. To proceed faster, to treat, or even to demonstrate the strokes out of sequence will bring about undesired reflex effects that will only frighten the patient and delay progress.[2] Although one must begin treatment carefully, one should also terminate all treatment with the basic and balancing strokes within the area treated.

Dicke lists and defines exact strokes and systematic treatments for various individual circumstances. Ebner also uses the case method approach, demonstrating the exact injury or disability and complete information that accompanies each case. This includes the patient's sex, age, and occupation, as well as Ebner's own examination and evaluation, and the patient's description of symptoms. A record of that which can be seen and felt, range of motion, pain, swelling in specific anatomical areas and treatment given, with exact notes of progress for each treatment is also included. Ebner, in certain instances, starts with the basic section and on the same day proceeds directly to the involved anatomical area of disability, unlike Dicke's strict adherence to the total system.

By studying Figure 24–1 one can see the areas of the back that Bindegewebsmassage relates to visceral problems, headache, etc. Begin with the basic strokes to the level of the disorder before concentrating on the strokes. Deviations from normal can be felt by the fingers, including tension, localized swelling, depressed areas, drawn-in bands of tissue, atrophy

---

[2]The author has found this to be true by experience.

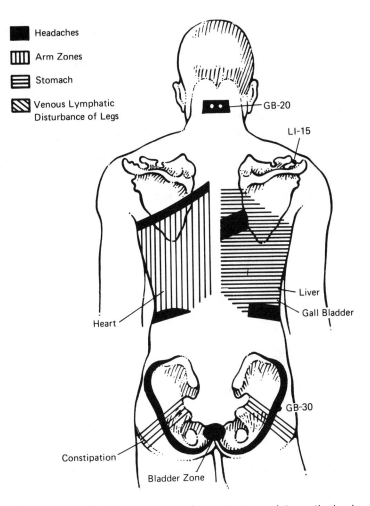

**Figure 24-1.** Some connective tissue zones and acupuncture points on the back.

of muscles or hypertrophy of muscles. Extreme tenderness in any involved area requires a very gentle approach leading gradually toward deeper pressure according to the patient's tolerance.

The patient should have no discomfort upon termination of the massage. Balancing strokes, and strokes treating the great trochanter or subcostal areas should return natural and comfortable sensations to the patient.

Dicke presents numerous disabilities that respond to this massage system, all of which are treated by the strokes described and illustrated here that follow segmental distribution upward on the spinal column to the level of enervation. Two principal types of pathologies respond especially well: changes in peripheral structures due to interference with their blood supply; and changes in peripheral structures occurring because of pathologic conditions related to other parts of the segmental distribution.

Dicke lists the following specific disabilities that respond well with Bindegewebsmassage treatment:

**Skin and under-skin.** symmetrical eczema, ichthyosis, itching skin, neurodermatitis, phlegmon, decubitus, scars

**Bones and joints.** fractures, orthopedic cases, periarthritis, epicondylitis, tendo-vaginitis, arthritis, arthrosis

**Musculature.** myalgia, lumbago, torticollis, progressive muscular dystrophy

**Nerves.** after treatment of neuritis, neuralgia, ischialgia, brachial neuralgia

**Blood and lymph vessels.** varicose symptoms complex, thrombophlebitis (subacute), hemorrhoids, edema

**Circulatory disturbances.** Raynaud's disease, Burger's disease, intermittent claudication, arteriosclerotic and diabetic gangrene, scleroderma, frostbite, tropic disturbances, Sudeck's atrophy

## Inner Organs

**Heart and circulatory diseases.** hypertonia, angina pectoris, myocardial dysfunctions, infarcts (subacute), functional disturbances

**Respiratory diseases.** bronchial asthma, chronic bronchitis, bronchiectasis, emphysema, postoperative situations

**Stomach diseases.** acute and chronic gastritis, ulcers, gastric atony, cardiospasms, functional disturbances

**Intestinal diseases.** spastic and atonic constipation, chronic colitis, colica mucosa, postoperative appendectomy

**Liver–gall bladder system diseases.** hepatitis (subacute), cholesystitis (subacute), postoperative gall bladder and bile duct operations

**Diseases of the kidneys and urinary systems.** nephritis and pyelitis postoperative and subacute conditions, enuresis nocturna

**Gynecological diseases.** infection of the ovaries and uterus (subacute and postoperative conditions)

**Endocrine disturbances.** amenorrhea, dysmenorrhea, lactation, genital infantilism, hyperthyroidism

**Central nervous system diseases.** after treatment of poliomyelitis, encephalitis, Little's disease, multiple sclerosis, Parkinson's disease

**Various headaches.** posttraumatic and rheumatic headache, migraines

**Sense organ diseases.** nose (cold), ears, eyes

**Allergies.** hay fever, bronchial asthma, eczema (of skin)

## Contraindications

These include tuberculosis at all stages, all malignant tumors, myoma, endometriosis, psychosis, and mental illnesses.

## HISTORY OF BINDEGEWEBSMASSAGE

Bindegewebsmassage was developed by Elisabeth Dicke of Germany, who, in 1929, suffered from a severe disturbance in the peripheral circulation of her right leg. As a result of a neglected tooth infection, a general toxemia developed, which resulted in an endarteritis obliterans of the right leg. This leg was cold and bluish in color, the toes giving the appearance of incipient gangrene. The dorsalis pedis artery was no longer palpable. Dicke was advised to consider amputation of the lower limb.

In addition to the extreme pain in the extremity, she suffered from an almost unbearable backache. While lying on her side she tried to give herself some relief by massaging over the painful areas of her back. She found that over the sacrum and the right iliac crest, thickenings and infiltrations could be palpated, and toward the left side on the same level, the skin felt tight.

She tried to ease the tension by massage with her fingers across the affected areas, but found that these areas were hypersensitive to touch. Slight stroking with the fingertip caused great pain. The tension, however, gradually subsided, the pain in the back eased, and an agreeable sensation of warmth took its place. On successive days she persisted with the stroking, with other people taking over the actual stroking. She gradually felt pins and needles in the affected leg, followed by a sensation of warmth.

In further treatments she incorporated the areas around the greater trochanter and along the iliotibial tract. Gradually the superficial venous circulation reappeared in the thigh and leg. The severe symptoms subsided after 3 more months of treatment carried out by a colleague under Dicke's direction. She was able to resume her occupation after a year.

Years of investigation followed. During the course of her illness, Dicke had experienced pathologic function of internal organs in addition to the symptoms in the back and leg. She suffered from a chronic gastritis, the liver showed enlargement, the heart showed symptoms of angina, and finally she experienced disturbance of kidney function. These visceral complaints cleared up simultaneously with the improvement of the peripheral circulation and normalization of the tissue changes in the back. Treatment of pathologically affected areas of the body surface helped to clear up pathologic changes in affected viscera. She discovered that certain areas on the body surface definitely related to certain viscera.

Systemic observation of patients in the following years confirmed these findings. Unknown to Dicke at the time, the English neurologist Head had already described similar findings, showing changes in the same well-defined areas of the body surface, pertaining to specific organs. These alterations appear when pathologic changes take place in affected viscera. These are known in the literature as "Head Zones" (*see* Chapter 20). The ancient Chinese, of course, became aware thousands of years ago of an increased sensitivity of certain skin areas (called points) when a body organ or function was impaired.

Further clinical investigations followed in 1938 under Kohlrausch and Tierich H. Leube in Freiburg, incorporating the basic work of J. MacKenzie. Head pointed out changes in skin areas, whereas MacKenzie (1917) drew attention to changes in muscle tone and sensitivity in areas sharing the same root supply with pathologically affected organs.[3]

Years of work and investigation resulted in the present-day method of Bindegewebsmassage in Germany. This method is now used in many other countries, being widely employed not only in pathologic conditions associated with visceral disease, but also in the treatment of diseases associated with the pathology of circulation. In this, it shows very gratifying results. In Germany, it is also widely used by members of the medical profession for diagnostic purposes.

## POSITION OF THE PATIENT

The patient may be in a sitting position for treatment; the patient may also be treated in a prone- or side-lying position.

## POSITION OF THE OPERATOR

As with other massage techniques, the operator should be in any position, be it seated or standing, that provides for good body mechanics and avoids fatigue.

## APPLICATION OF TECHNIQUE

Using the pad of the middle finger, touch the patient's skin very firmly without applying more pressure than is necessary. Fingernails must be very short. The strokes must be applied with even pressure and speed.

---

[3]Ebner (1962), p. 3.

## GENERAL PRINCIPLES

Each stroke is done three times. The right side is done first, then the left side. Loss of hand contact occurs with completion of each stroke. The hand that is not working is kept in touch with the patient at all times. Use the third fingertip and let the fourth finger follow. Get your pull through the entire arm. Feel for spinal and pelvic bony structures and follow their edges. *Use no lubricant.*

Flat strokes are done by using more finger area and a lighter stroke. Steep strokes are done with less finger area and deeper pressure. Exploration of the body tissues will reveal tightness in certain areas, as well as flattened or drawn areas. The fingers applying pressure will often "skip" when they encounter such areas. Localized swelling can be felt. Atrophy or hypertrophy of muscles can be noticed. Even bony deformities can at times be felt. Mobility of the layers of connective tissue can be evaluated. Painful areas can be assessed. Palpation of the muscles will give information as to the degree of tension present. Any asymmetry or muscle imbalance can be felt.

Grip the tissues between the thumb and fingers, lifting them away from the superficial layer. In some areas it may be impossible to lift the tissues if they are tight or painful. This usually indicates a pathologic condition. (Fig. 24–1 shows reflex areas on the back that relate to visceral pathologies as discovered by Head and MacKenzie.) There are also areas on the back that relate to headache, constipation, arterial disease of the legs, and venous lymphatic disorders of the legs. Drawn-in areas over the scapula and posterior deltoid indicate disorders of the upper extremity.

By pulling from the fifth lumbar vertebrae to the occiput, first on one side of the spine, then on the other, abnormal areas will become red or even raise a wheal. The spinal level can indicate areas of involvement. This is called the diagnostic stroke. Care must be taken that the pressure of this stroke is not painfully deep. The third finger leads and the fourth finger follows. The angle of the strokes is between 40 and 60 degrees. *Pull*, do not *push*, the tissues under the fingers.

Uncomfortable feelings may be reported by the patient, including a cutting or a scratching sensation, or a feeling of dull pressure. This indicates a pathologic condition. If the fingers find it hard to "pull through" tight areas, they should not be forced. Depending on body build, age, and other normal conditions of the body, some deviations occur in every normal human being. All findings should be indicated in writing on a chart or diagram. Progress should also be recorded.

## Direction of Strokes

In the paravertebral areas the stroke follows the direction of the dermatomes. In the periphery it follows the direction of the muscle fibers, muscle, fascia, tendons, or at right angles to facial borders.

## Procedures for Treatment

The back is divided into three sections, the basic section, the thoracic section, and the cervical section. The basic section *(grundaufbau)* includes the coccyx through the first lumbar vertebrae. No treatment is ever given without covering the basic section with a build up of the back strokes to the level of the part of the body involved; in cases of the upper extremity, all three parts precede local treatment.

## Precautions

Adverse effects such as nausea, dizziness, fainting, diarrhea, and profuse perspiration may result if treatment is too harsh or done improperly. The person giving the massage should watch the patient intently; should any of the above become apparent, balancing strokes should be done immediately.

## BALANCING STROKES

For thoracic balancing strokes, the patient should be standing. Stroke with flat, gentle fingers on the right side three times. From T-12, follow the lower border of the last rib, around the chest, to the mammillary line, pulling very gently, lifting the tissue slightly at the end of the stroke. Repeat this same technique three times on the left.

The five pectoral balancing strokes are as follows: (1) from the middle third of the sternum to the axillary line; (2) from the middle third of the sternum to a little above the end of the first stroke; (3) from the upper third of the sternum to the capsule of the shoulder; (4) from the top of the sternum to the lower border of the clavicle; and (5) out to the capsule of the shoulder. Repeat this technique until the series of five strokes are done three times, first on the right side and then repeated on the left side.

The *great balancing stroke* goes from C-7 to the coccyx. A flat bilateral stroke is done down the erector spinae group to L-5, where the hands separate and follow the line of the rhombus to the posterior inferior spine of the ilium. Then, continue diagonally downward to the anal fold and coccyx. Repeat this technique three times (Figs. 24–2 and 24–3).

## BASIC TREATMENT (GRUNDAUFBAU)

### From Coccyx Through L-1

Stroke from the posterior inferior spine of the ilium downward to the coccyx on the right side three times. Repeat on the left. These strokes may be steep unless tension causes pain or other adverse effects.

These strokes are followed by strokes from the posterior inferior spine of the ilium upward to L-5. The stroke ends in a "hook-on"; first on the right side three times, then on the left. A hook-on is frequently used to complete

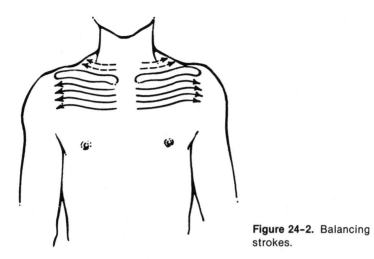

**Figure 24-2.** Balancing strokes.

a stroke. The fingers make a comma-shaped, short, deep stroke at the end of the longer stroke.

Next, give three pelvis strokes on the right side. Follow the crest of the ilium, from L-5 around the pelvis to the anterior superior iliac spine. Finish the stroke with a light pulling up of the tissue. Repeat three times. Then, stroke from the posterior inferior spine of the ilium around the pelvis to the anterior superior iliac spine. Finish with a light pulling up of the tissue.

Now, stroke from the anal fold. Stroke behind and under the tuberosity of the ischium around the greater trochanter of the femur and below it, over the tensor fascia lata, then upward in front to the anterior superior iliac spine. Repeat this on the left side.

After this, give a series of hook-ons. Start on the right side and go around with five little hook-ons from L-5 to L-1, the first hook-on, L-5 to L-4, beginning on the medial border of the erector spinae, ending at spinous process; continue to L-1. Alternate these strokes right and left until each side has been done three times.

The fan strokes are flat, soft pulls, diagonally downward, in an area between an imaginary line from the highest point on the pelvic crest to the L-3. Each stroke ends in the lumbosacral joint. Alternate the entire fan stroke right and left, until done three times on both sides (Fig. 24–4).

From the basic strokes the system moves upwards along the vertebral column.

## From T-12 to T-7

The person giving the massage should be standing. Administer five hook-on strokes that proceed from T-12 to T-7, alternating from right to left. Repeat this series three times.

Continue with intercostal strokes, seven gentle ascending strokes begin-

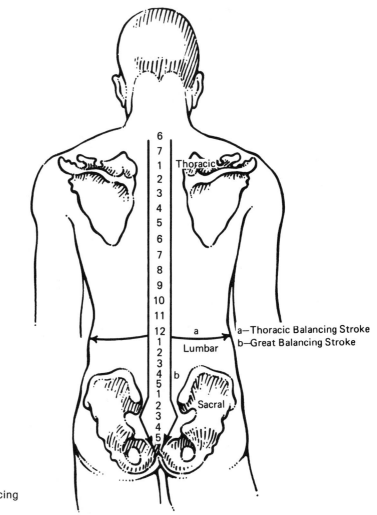

**Figure 24-3.** Balancing strokes.

ning over the lowest rib from the posterior border of the anterior axillary line. Each stroke ends with a small hook-on on the vertebrae from T-12 to T-6.

The seven additional strokes are used only in special treatment for chest conditions. They are the exact reverse of the preceding intercostal strokes.

Pectoral balance strokes, as previously described, are done at this point. Add two strokes that follow the superior border of the clavicle, going from medial to lateral (*see* Fig. 24-2).

The next section of strokes goes from T-7 to C-7. Start and finish on the right. Proceed to the left only if treating both sides. With heart disease do not treat the left side. Usually only one shoulder is treated.

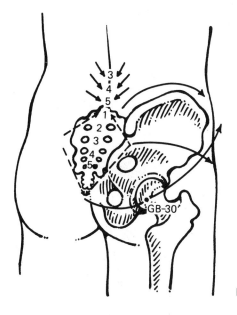

**Figure 24-4.** Basic strokes.

Then, treat the upper extremity in the following steps. Beginning on the right side, do gentle hook-ons from T-7 to C-7 alternating to the left side, three times on each side. Stroke from the vertebral column to the scapula with five strokes beginning from T-7 to the inferior angle of the scapula, working upward and finishing each stroke with a hook-on under the scapula. If swelling is found, do not treat above that level. Pull from the inferior angle of the scapula upward, following *under* the scapula's spinal border to the level of the spine of the scapula three times, using steep strokes. With a flat, gentle stroke, follow the axillary border of the scapula over the teres major. Be gentle when approaching the axillary region. Stay above the axillary line. With the heel of the hand on the shoulder (with bent fingers) follow the superior aspect of the spine of the scapula from the vertebrae to the axillary aspect of the scapula. This is a pivot-like stroke (Fig. 24–5).

To accomplish widening of the shoulder joint, brace the hypothenar eminence of the hand near the border of the latissimus dorsi. Have fingers reach under the tendon of the latissimus dorsi and pull by flexing the fingers in the palm. While standing and holding the tissues with one hand, stroke the latissimus dorsi *toward* the insertion with a short stroke upward. Stretch the pectorals pulling from the inferior angle of the scapula to the tendon of the pectorals.

Prepare for the next strokes with short, little friction, circular strokes, first on the latissimus tendon, then on the pectorals. Standing at the side of the patient, tuck each hand into one side of the armpit. "Widen" the joint by letting the hands fall open, stretching the pectorals and the latissimus dorsi.

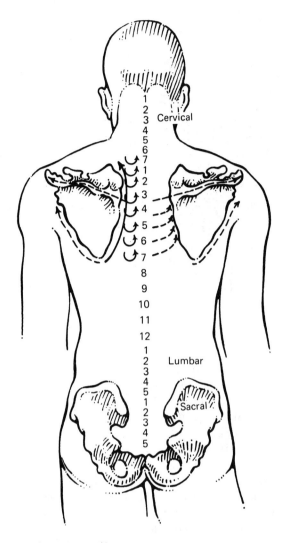

Note: Not All Strokes Are Illustrated Bilaterally.
Follow Written Instructions.

**Figure 24-5.** Pivot-like strokes.

From the inferior angle of the scapula, stroke back toward the scapula to the ventral aspect of the axillary border, stretching the latissimus tendon and stroking over the serratus anterior. Alternate with similar strokes in a reverse direction to stretch the pectorals at the end of the stroke. Crossing the hands, alternately stroke toward the latissimus dorsi, then toward the pectorals. Support the lower trapezius with the left hand and stroke toward the shoulder (Figs. 24–6 and 24–7).

The next section goes from C-7 to C-1. The "sun stroke" (Fig. 24-8), in

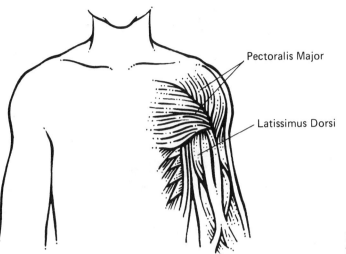

Pectoralis Major

Latissimus Dorsi

**Figure 24-6.** Widening of the shoulder joint.

five short strokes that begin on a diagonal, strokes toward C-7. Begin on the lower right side working toward the top right side of C-7.

Ascend from C-7 through C-1 with a light pull along the side of the spinous processes (Fig. 24–9). Alternate right to left three times. Administer hook-ons from C-7 to C-1.

Be sure to stabilize the head with the opposing hand alternating right to left three times. Stroke straight across the nuchal line three times in each direction (Fig. 24–9). Pectoral balancing may be included, if necessary, on the lower rhombus strokes for balance (*see* Fig. 24–2). Give an ascending small stroke along the anterior upper two thirds of the right trapezius to its origin. Lightly outline the right sternocleidomastoid, staying on the posterior border from its origin up to its insertion on the mastoid bone (Fig. 24–10).

Repeat on the left side three times. Using both hands stroke from the anterior trapezius across it. This is a bilateral small stroke that pulls across the ascending trapezius to just below C-7. This is a balancing stroke (*see* Figs. 24–2, 24–3). Use a final balancing stroke from C-7 to the coccyx as previously described.

## Treatment for Chest

Asthma may be made worse if this technique is not done exactly right. The person giving the treatment should be standing. Do all the basic strokes followed by the thoracic build-up if the patient will tolerate it. Otherwise, do only the basic strokes until the patient can tolerate the treatment. Add strokes in the reverse direction of the intercostal strokes. Do the right side first, then the left, alternating three times between sides, finishing on the right side. Continue with cross strokes from the right to the left and left to

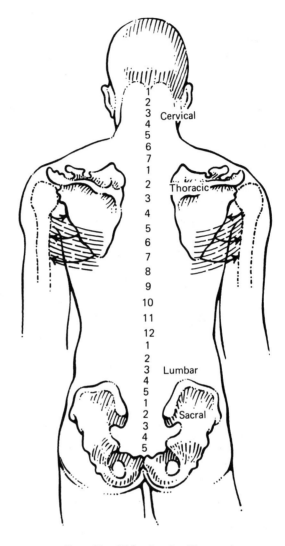

Cervical

Thoracic

Lumbar

Sacral

Note: Not All Strokes Are Illustrated.

**Figure 24-7.** Widening of the shoulder joint.

right between the scapula up to the spine of the scapula (Fig 24–11). Do widening of the shoulder joint (*see* Figs. 24–6 and 24–7).

Give intercostal strokes toward the sternum from the posterior axillary line. Do four strokes, repeating the last one in the same place. Provide a long stroke the length of the sternum from the zyphoid upward to the interclavicular ligament. Give hook-ons to the sternum, first on the right and then on the left, alternating sides. Do short, flat strokes to the sternocleidomastoid insertion. Then use short strokes between the clavicles over the interclavicular ligament proceeding across the manubrium. Pectoral bal-

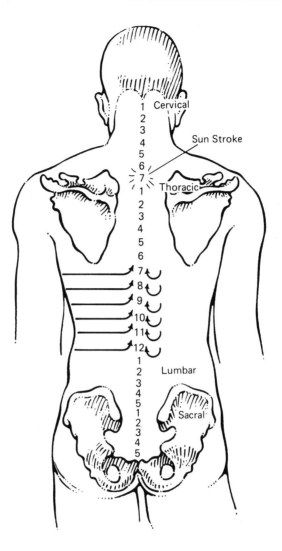

Note: All of the Following Represent "Hook On" Strokes

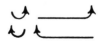

**Figure 24-8.** Rib strokes and hook-ons, T-12 to T-7 sun stroke.

ance strokes should be included for the benefit of the patient (*see* Fig. 24–2).

Strokes across the sternum from its lower end upwards, working across the manubrium, should be administered next. Pectoral strokes are done as a treatment stroke with hook-ons at the end of the stroke (*see* Fig. 24–10).

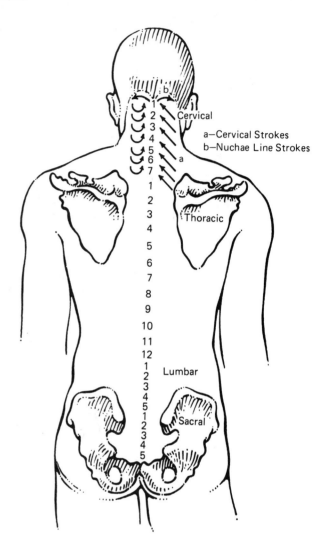

**Figure 24-9.** Upper back strokes C-7 to C-1.

The pectoral stroke is done as a balance stroke. Provide a long stroke from the twelfth rib up to C-7.

## Wrist, Hand and Fingers

With the exception of stroking from proximal to distal, Dicke's strokes cover the hand completely. This author prefers most massage strokes to proceed from distal to proximal.

To perform these strokes, the operator uses the soft pads of the middle finger, pulling with some depth from proximal to distal. Both thumbs rest on the patient's wrist with no pressure during these strokes.

All strokes previously described can be adapted to these smaller areas and must be mastered.

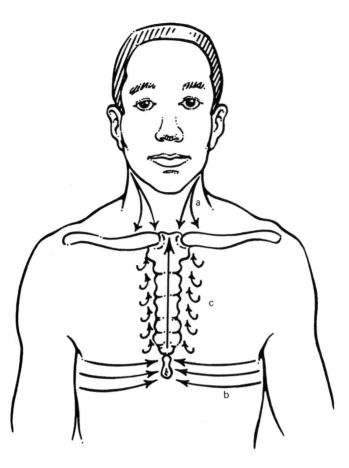

Note: Not All Strokes Are Illustrated; Please Follow the
Written Instructions.

**Figure 24-10.** Treatment for the chest, anterior.

As illustrated in Figure 24–13a, the first stroke pulls over the lower third of the flexor carpi radialis. The second stroke pulls over the palmaris longus (Fig. 24–13b). The third stroke pulls over the flexor carpi ulnaris (Fig. 24–13c).

These are followed by short strokes over the volar ligament. Be careful not to press too deeply over the median nerve. Stabilize above the wrist. Get the pull by flexing the fingers. Start on the radial side and work toward the ulnar side (Fig. 24–14).

Next, follow with short strokes over the transverse ligament across the heel of the hand from thenar to hypothenar eminences (Fig 24–15a). Then long strokes are done over the palmar fascia, working deep to the interossei, pulling toward the fingers (Fig. 24–15b). Thenar strokes, which are half

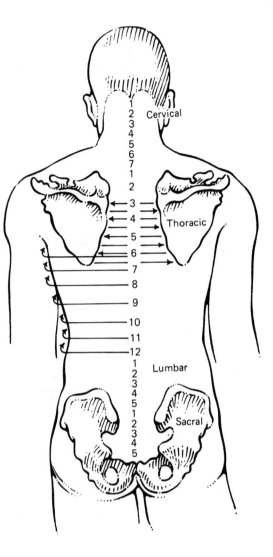

**Figure 24-11.** Treatment for the chest, posterior.

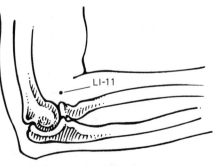

**Figure 24-12.** Elbow and forearm.

LI-11 — Chu-chih

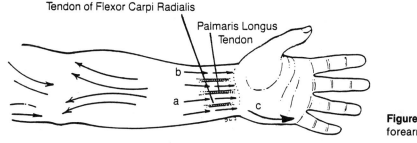

Tendon of Flexor Carpi Radialis

Palmaris Longus
Tendon

**Figure 24-13.** Elbow and forearm.

ellipsoid, are then given over the inner surface of the thenar eminence (Fig. 24–15c).

Transverse strokes are then done over the thenar eminence, working from the inner border outward toward the dorsal surface (Fig. 24–16a). Hypothenar strokes of a similar nature are done in a longitudinal direction (Fig. 24–16b) and in a transverse direction (Fig. 24–16c).

Small, interdigit, longitudinal strokes over the transverse palmaris ligament between the heads of the metacarpals should then be done (Fig. 24–17).

On the dorsum of the hand, short strokes should be done. Anchor the thumb on the volar side. Start radially over the ligamentum dorsalis, and go distally across the ligament adding gentle, passive extension of the wrist simultaneously (Fig. 24–18a).

Next, perform long, flat gentle strokes over the interossei (Fig. 24–18b).

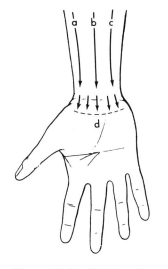

**Figure 24-14.** Stroking the palmaris longus.

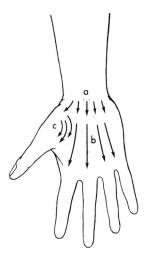

**Figure 24-15.** Stroking the hand.

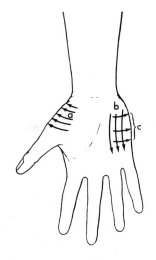

**Figure 24-16.** Transverse and hypothenar strokes of the hand.

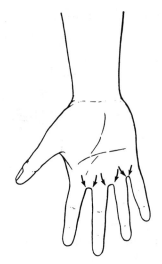

**Figure 24-17.** Longitudinal strokes over the transverse palmaris ligament.

The following stroke is best done with the thumbs. It is a pull and counterpull to stretch the web between the fingers. One hand holds, while the other pulls the next finger away, providing gentle passive motion as well as stroking. Begin on the radial side and work toward the ulnar side. This

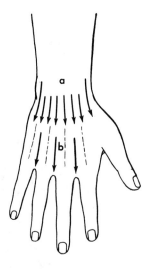

**Figure 24-18.** Strokes over the transverse palmaris ligament, the interossei, and the dorsum of the hand.

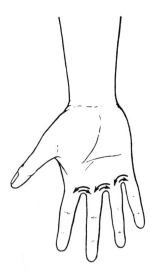

**Figure 24-19.** Pulling stroke over the fingers.

should be done to both the volar and the dorsal surfaces of the hand (Figs. 24–19 and 24–20).

## Massage of the Fingers

Each finger should be massaged before going on to the next one.

Pull out the long tendons on the volar side of the fingers, stroking the tendon from metacarpophalangeal joint to the tip of the finger. Use one hand to support the patient's hand, to prevent hyperextension of the finger, and to get the proper pressure. *This pulling is not done by grasping the finger, but by stroking along the tendon* (Fig. 24–21a). Next, perform small strokes on the medial and lateral borders of the first two phalanges (Fig. 24–21b). Follow this by stroking, proximal to distal, with a *little* stretch, over the collateral ligaments of each joint. *Do not pull* into the joint space or go beyond one joint at a time (Fig. 24–21c). Stretching of the small joints can be done (Fig. 24–21d).

Stretch each joint of each finger by using both thumbs on the dorsal side and both third fingers, pulling outward (Fig. 24–22).

Next, apply short strokes over the dorsal aponeurosis, beginning on the thumb. Stretch the long extensor tendons between each joint (Fig. 24–23). If the lumbercales are involved, stroke laterally between each joint.

Stretch the palmar fascia in the following fashion. With the thumbs on the dorsum of the patient's hand, the operator pronates his or her own hands, stretching the palm of the patient's hand. The volar aspect of the patient's hand is supported by the hypothenar aspect of the operator's hand. Start at the carpal area and work distally with each stroke (Fig. 24–24).

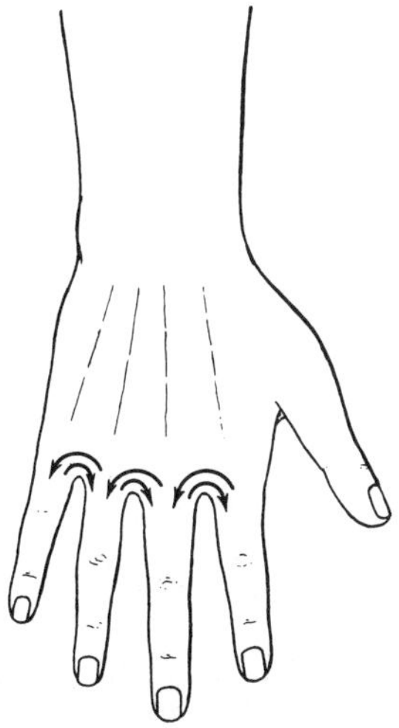

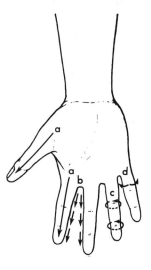

**Figure 24-20.** Counterpull.

**Figure 24-21.** Massage of the fingers.

**Figure 24-22** Stretching the finger joints.

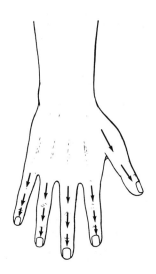

**Figure 24-23.** Stretching the finger joints.

Although Dicke would not do so, this author recommends stroking off the entire extremity with effleurage, working from firm pressure gradually toward lighter pressure, and finishing with light effleurage strokes that follow the venous flow.

### Lower Extremity

Precede treatment of the leg with the basic treatment, with the patient, if possible, in a seated position. Next, ask the patient to lie in a supine posi-

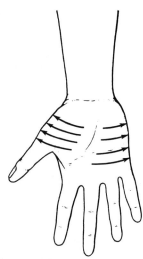

**Figure 24-24.** Stretching the palmar fascia.

tion. Face the patient and always stabilize the patient's leg with the free hand. As before, all strokes are done three times.

Then commence with the following strokes. From the superior dorsal border of the greater trochanter follow the iliotibial band, ending the stroke over the insertion of the lateral hamstring with a hook-on (Fig. 24–25). Facing the head of the patient, surround the greater trochanter with small ellipsoid strokes. Beginning distally, follow the iliotibial band for its upper two-thirds and finish the stroke around the greater trochanter. Give ellipsoid strokes in the space between the greater trochanter up to the iliac spine. Support the leg with the free hand from the lateral side. Stroke between the semi-membranosis and the semi-tendinosis down the lower third with a stretch hook-on technique at the end of the stroke, near its insertion (Fig. 24–26).

Bimanually stroke both hamstrings from the gluteal fold to their distal portion, where the hands are turned outward at the end of the stroke to provide a stretch of the tendons at their insertion. (Never use this stroke if varicosity exists.) Stroke from the distal gastrocnemius where the belly begins to the knee, turning the hands outward at the top of the gastrocnemius. This movement comes through the arms, not the fingers. Stay in the groove, stroking gently. Provide widening of the knee by using both hands to provide a bilateral stretch or widening technique to the popliteal space, stretching first the hamstrings then the gastrocnemius (Fig. 24–27).

## Lower Extremity and Foot

Bimanually, stroke the Achilles tendon, working from proximal to distal, beginning just distal to the belly of the muscle, pulling to the back of the heel. The hand should help to flex the foot slightly. Stroke the peroneous longus and brevis, around the malleolus toward the dorsum of the foot. Stabilize the leg with the other hand. Do the same for the posterior tibialis. Bimanually, stroke down both sides. (Figure 24–28 illustrates a posterior view of these strokes; Figure 24–29 illustrates the lateral view of the above strokes; and Figure 24–30, the medial view.)

If arthritis is present in the knee, do not do the following strokes. Face the patient. With one hand, use short strokes that hook under the border of the patella, while stabilizing the patient's leg with the other hand. Begin

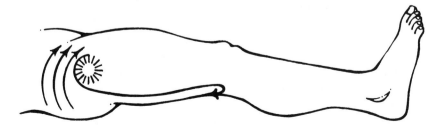

**Figure 24–25.** Lower extremity.

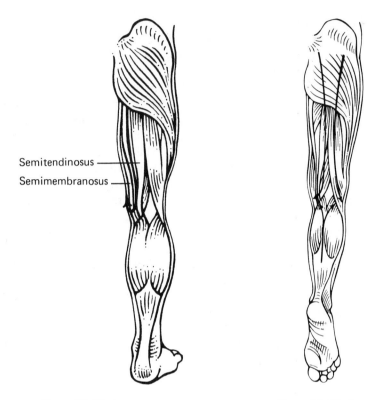

Semitendinosus
Semimembranosus

**Figure 24-26.** Lower extremity.

**Figure 24-27.** Lower extremity and foot.

medially and work to the lateral knee. The finger should be bent, trying to reach under the patella. First, do the superior aspect of the patella; then stroke around the inferior aspect of the patella, stroking toward it using the other hand and using a pivot-like stroke in which the heel of the hand acts as the pivot to stroke around the patella. Stroke across the top of the patella from medial to lateral. Then below, stroke from the medial to the lateral aspect (Fig. 24–31). Stabilizing the foot with one hand, apply little strokes across the front of the ankle joint, dorsi flexing the ankle at the same time. Provide short little strokes between the metatarsophalangeal joints, proximal to distal, medial to lateral. The dorsum of the foot is not treated. Apply deep little strokes just in front of the heel from the arch around the side of the foot, always starting laterally and working medially. Do the same to the medial side of the foot, going the other way around. Then give short strokes across the heel (Figs. 24–32 and 24–33).

Provide deep stroking of the plantar aspect of the foot with long strokes covering the longitudinal arch from the heel up to the metatarsophalangeal joint. Then stroke the lateral and medial borders of the foot. Repeat this on

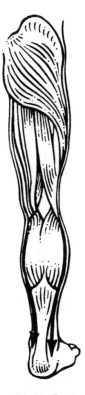

**Figure 24-28.** Posterior view, lower extremity and foot.

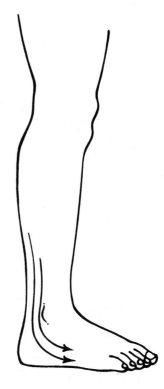

**Figure 24-29.** Lateral view, lower extremity and foot.

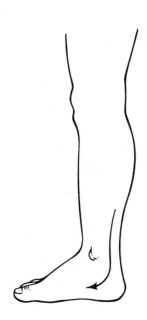

**Figure 24-30.** Medial view, lower extremity and foot.

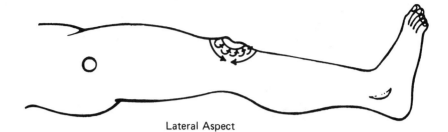

Lateral Aspect

**Figure 24-31.** Pivot-like strokes to the patella.

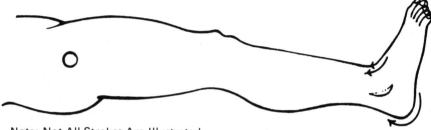

Note: Not All Strokes Are Illustrated.

**Figure 24-32.** Foot, lateral view.

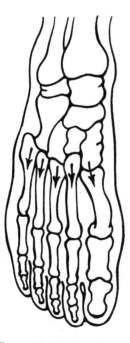

**Figure 24-33.** Foot, frontal view.

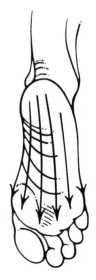

**Figure 24-34.** Stretching the foot.

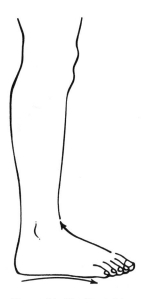

**Figure 24-35.** Stretching the foot.

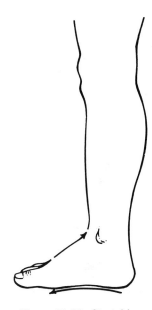

**Figure 24-36.** Stretching the foot.

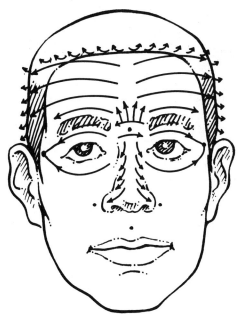

**Figure 24-37.** Face, frontal view.

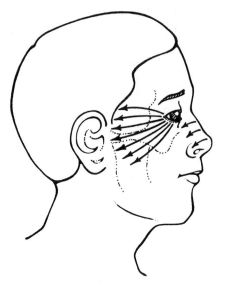

**Figure 24-38.** Face, lateral view.

**TABLE 24-1. A COMPARISON OF BINDEGEWEBSMASSAGE AND ACUPUNCTURE POINTS**

| Acupuncture Point | Anatomical Site | Disabilities |
|---|---|---|
| B-40 | At the center of the popliteal fossa | Knee pain |
| B-60 | Midpoint between the posterior margin of the lateral malleolus and the Achilles tendon | Diseases of the ankle joint and surrounding soft tissue |
| GB-20 | Midpoint of a line joining the tip of the mastoid process to the posterior midline in the groove between the trapezius and the sternocleidomastoid | Headache Hypertension |
| GB-21 | Midway between C-7 and acromion process | Shoulder and back pain Upper extremity impairment |
| GB-30 | One-third of the distance from the greater trochanter to the base of the coccyx | Lower extremity circulatory disorders |
| GB-34 | Anterior to the neck of the fibula | Lower extremity disorders Knee pain |
| LI-11 | Radial end of fold of fully flexed elbow | Disorders of the elbow joint and surrounding soft tissue |
| LI-15 | In the depression of the acromion in the center of the deltoid muscle when the arm is abducted to 90° | Pain and impaired movement of elbow and arm. Disorders of the shoulder and surrounding soft tissue |
| Special Point 1 Yin-tang | At the glabella, midway between the medial margins of the eyebrows | Disorders of the nose Headache |
| Special Point 2 Tai-yang | At the temple, one cun directly posterior to the midpoint of a line joining the lateral canthus of the eye and the lateral margin of the eyebrow | Facial paralysis |

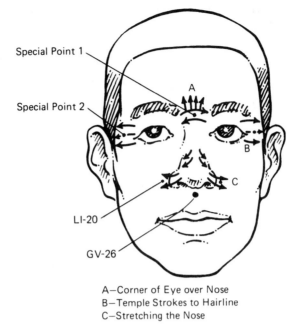

A—Corner of Eye over Nose
B—Temple Strokes to Hairline
C—Stretching the Nose

**Figure 24-39.** Comparison of acupuncture points and anatomical sites used in Bindegewebs-massage. Frontal view of face.

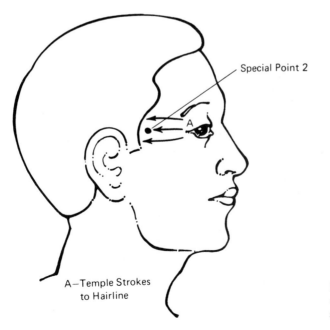

A—Temple Strokes to Hairline

**Figure 24-40.** Lateral view of face showing temple strokes to hairline.

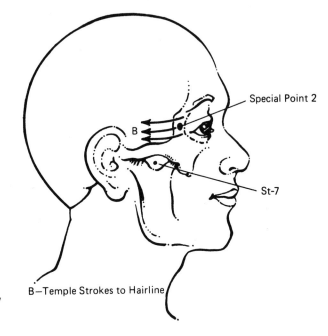

**Figure 24-41.** Lateral view of face.

Special Point 2

B

St-7

B—Temple Strokes to Hairline

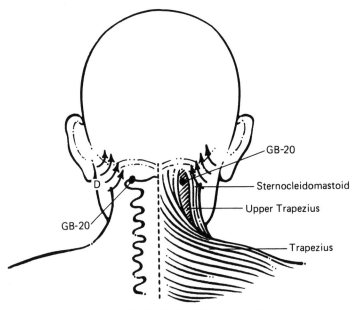

GB-20

Sternocleidomastoid

Upper Trapezius

Trapezius

D

GB-20

D—Stroke on Posterior Skull along Ligamentum Nuchae to Mastoid Process

**Figure 24-42.** Back and neck.

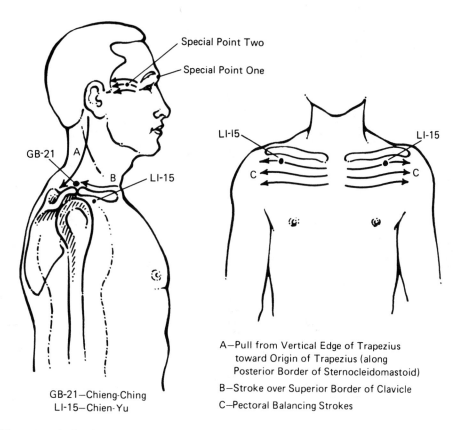

A—Pull from Vertical Edge of Trapezius
   toward Origin of Trapezius (along
   Posterior Border of Sternocleidomastoid)

B—Stroke over Superior Border of Clavicle

C—Pectoral Balancing Strokes

GB-21—Chieng-Ching
LI-15—Chien-Yu

**Figure 24-43.** Back and neck.

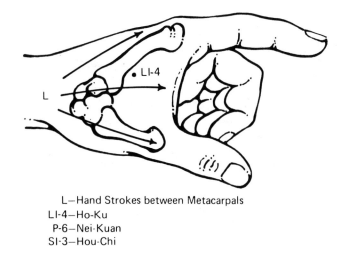

L—Hand Strokes between Metacarpals
LI-4—Ho-Ku
P-6—Nei-Kuan
SI-3—Hou-Chi

**Figure 24-44.** Hand.

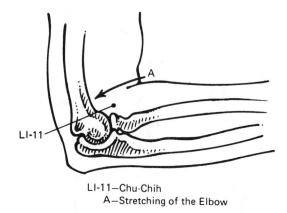

LI-11—Chu-Chih
A—Stretching of the Elbow

**Figure 24-45.** Elbow.

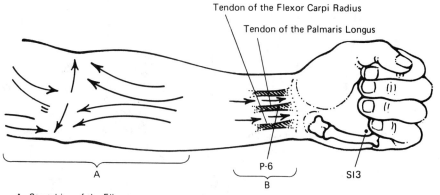

A—Stretching of the Elbow
B—Strokes over the Flexor Carpi Radius,
   Palmaris Longus, and Flexor Carpi Ulnaris

**Figure 24-46.** Forearm.

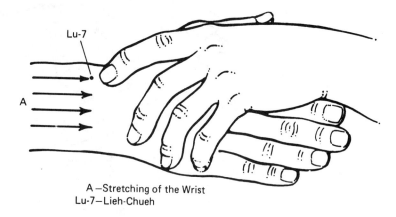

A—Stretching of the Wrist
Lu-7—Lieh-Chueh

**Figure 24-47.** Wrist.

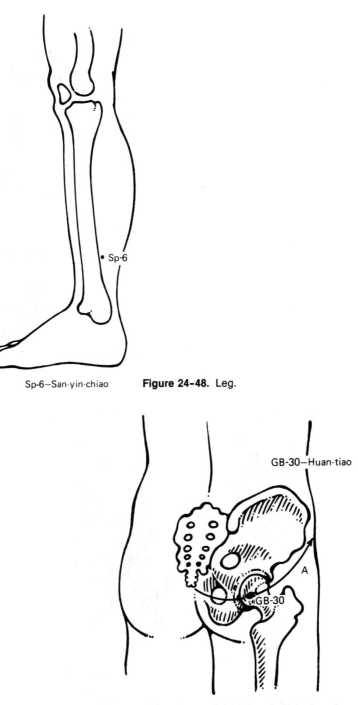

Sp-6—San-yin-chiao        **Figure 24-48.** Leg.

GB-30—Huan-tiao

A

GB-30

A—Pelvic stroke from anal fold along ischial tuberosity

**Figure 24-49.** Pelvic stroke.

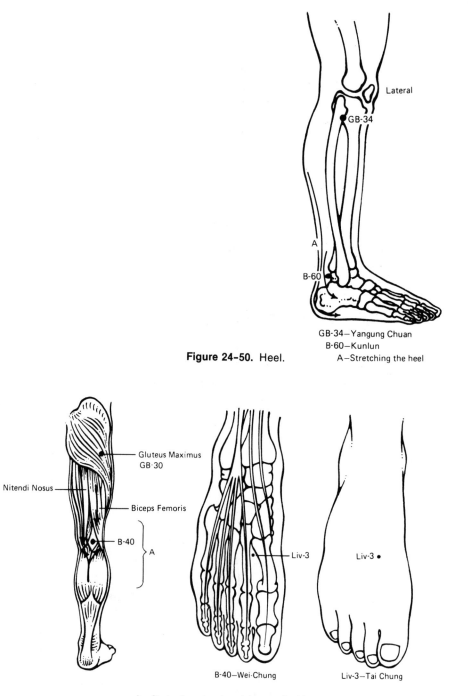

GB-34—Yangung Chuan
B-60—Kunlun
A—Stretching the heel

**Figure 24-50.** Heel.

A —Strokes from dorsal seat fold to popliteal fossa
and strokes along gastrocnemius into popliteal fossa

B-40—Wei-Chung          Liv-3—Tai Chung

**Figure 24-51.** Leg and foot.

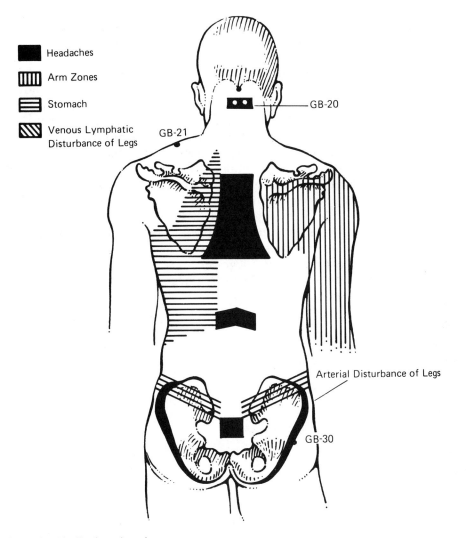

**Figure 24-52.** Back and neck.

the lateral aspect of the plantar surface. Apply medial plantar stroking across the muscle fibers at a right angle to the longitudinal arch.

Bilaterally stretch both the top and the bottom of the foot with a rolling motion of the hands. Go up and out on the proximal part of the foot. Pronate the hands with pressure and continue the same technique to the distal part of the foot. Then supinate the hands and forearms (Figs. 24–34 to 24–36).

**Face**

Stand behind the patient so that the patient's head leans against the operator. Using bimanual strokes across the forehead, stroke three times from the hairline until just above the eyebrows, moving towards the temple.

Short hook-on strokes from the midline to the temple, starting on the involved side are given. Do all of one side of the face and then the other.

Give very soft pulls into the hairline of the temple from the lateral side of the eye. Have your hand well anchored. Follow the upper eyebrow, stroking medial to lateral to the temple. Repeat the same, following the lower rim of the eyebrow. Give similar strokes just below the eye. Give short strokes upward between the eyes. Pull from the involved side to the other side over the bridge of the nose. Give "bimanual" widening of the nose by stroking from the center to each side. Bimanually stroke over the zygotmaticus working from just under the eyes toward the mandible, stroking from the front to the back with four strokes (Figs. 24–37, 24–38). Finish with the balancing stroke down the back.

Table 24–1 and Figures 24–39 to 24–52 compare acupuncture points and overlapping anatomical sites used in the Bindegewebsmassage system that claim relief of symptoms for the same disabilities. A careful study in which areas treated with Bindegewebsmassage are compared with acupuncture as done by the Japanese and Chinese seems to confirm the relationship between the two systems.

# — 25

# Reflexology

Although acupuncture is seldom given on the bottom of the foot, the Chinese feel that the total body is reflected in the ear, the eye, the palm of the hand, and the bottom of the foot. A great deal of emphasis has been placed on treating disorders of the entire body by treating the bottom of the foot with rather deep pressure in certain key spots.

Centuries before Head identified viscerocutaneous and cutaneovisceral reflex effects in the 1800s, the Chinese had identified sensitive areas on the bottom of the feet. Using finger pressure because needles were too painful, they treated specific areas on the feet to normalize physiologic functions in the human body.

William H. Fitzgerald rediscovered this Chinese method of foot massage and brought it to the attention of the medical world in the United States in 1913, calling it "Zone Therapy." It continues to be taught by descendants of Eunice D. Ingham, a major advocate of this technique.[1]

The technique for administration of this form of massage consists of compression, using the thumbs to apply firm pressure. By doing compression over the entire foot, tender areas will indicate where concentration of treatment should be given. Twenty minutes is an adequate amount of time to treat both feet. Care should be taken to stay within the patient's pain

---

[1] The purpose of this discussion is to bring Zone therapy to the attention of the reader. For greater detail, consult Eunice D. Ingham. (1959). *Stories the feet can tell*. Rochester, NY: Eunice D. Ingham.

The illustrations used here are not those from Ingham's text, but are adapted from *The massage book* by George Downing, illustrated by Anne Kent Rush (1974). New York: Random House; Berkeley, CA: The Bookworks, pp. 151–152.

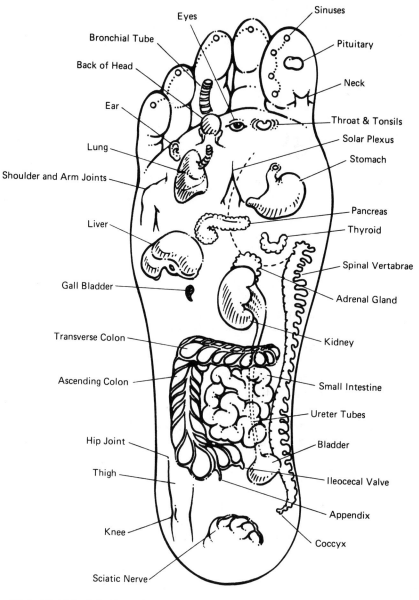

**Figure 25-1.** Right foot, bottom view.

tolerance level. The one being treated should be told that pressure needs to be firm but not overly painful.

Skilled and experienced thumbs can palpate areas of tightness or swelling on the foot. All references concerning Zone therapy agree as to which areas relate to various parts of the body. Attempts to explain physiologi-

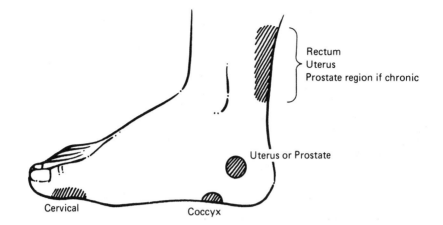

**Figure 25-2.** Right foot, lateral view.

cally why Zone therapy is effective are as difficult as explaining any of the other methods referred to in this text. The term *energy flow* in the human body is often used in recent research findings to describe such phenomena (*see* Chapter 5).

The palm of the hand can also be used and is sometimes easier for those who are knowledgeable and wish to treat themselves (*see* Fig. 25-4).

Other massage systems maintain that the connective tissue and the lymph system throughout the body are the vehicles for energy circuits of a

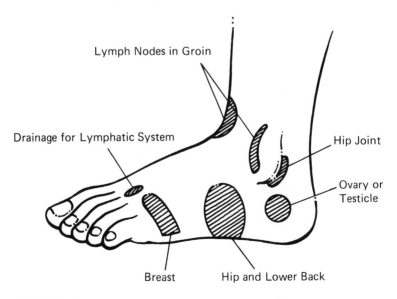

**Figure 25-3.** Left foot.

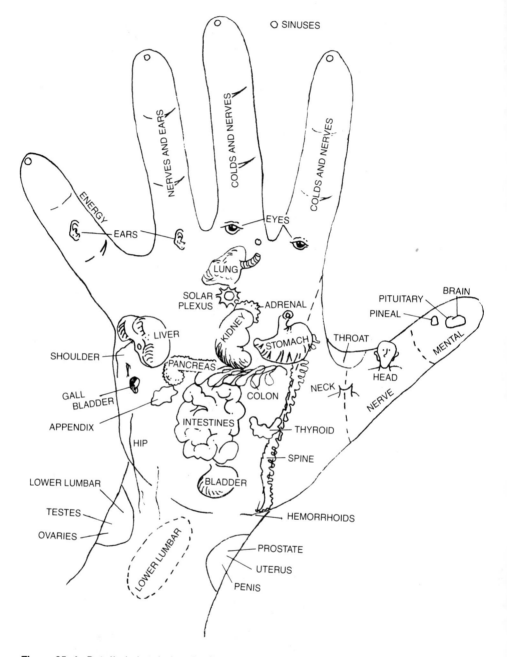

**Figure 25-4.** Detailed sketch, hand reflexology, right hand.

nature not yet analyzed by either Eastern or Western medical science. It is the author's belief that when the explanation is found for the effects of acupuncture, the foundations for the physiologic effects of Zone therapy and Bindegewebsmassage (connective tissue massage) will also be discovered.

## SUMMARY

Although this discussion is brief, the explanation plus the illustrations give the reader an idea of the procedures. It is recommended, however, that further course work on this topic be undertaken if the operator intends to become skillful in the use of reflexology.

# — 26

# James Cyriax

James Cyriax thinks that the most potent form of massage is deep friction:

> The principle governing the treatment of muscles during the acute or chronic stage is the same. The endeavor must be to prevent the continued adherence of unwanted young fibrous tissue in recent cases, or to rupture adherent scar tissue in long-standing cases. To stretch out a muscle does not widen the distance between its fibres; on the contrary, during stretching they lie more closely. Whereas, then, for the rupture of adherent scars about a joint, forced movement is required; interfibrillary adhesions in muscle can be broken, not by stretching, but by forcibly broadening the muscle out. Particularly is this true of the fibres of attachment of muscle into bone, where the vicinity of stationary tissue restricts the mobility of adjacent muscle. *Thus, deep transverse frictions restore mobility to muscle in the same way a manipulation frees a joint. Indeed, the action of deep transverse friction may be summed up as affording a mobilization that passive stretching or active exercises cannot achieve.*
>
> After the friction has restored a full range of painless broadening to the muscle belly, this added mobility must be maintained. To this end, the patient should perform a series of active contractions with the joint placed in a position that fully relaxes the affected muscle, i.e., the position that allows the greatest broadening. Strong resisted movements should be avoided until the scar has consolidated itself; otherwise, started too soon, they tend to strain the healing breach again. Athletes in particular must be careful to return to full sport with proper timing.[1]

---

[1]James Cyriax & Gillean Russell. (1977). *Textbook of orthopaedic medicine, Vol. II* (9th ed.). London: Bailliere Tindall. (Distributed by Macmillan, New York.)

## TYPES OF MANUAL TREATMENT

### Deep Effleurage

This technique serves to relieve congestion. Swelling is treated in many situations by upward stroking of sufficient depth to remove it. The chief indications for effleurage are oedema and traumatic periostitis.

### Oedema

Whether the oedema appears as the result of an injury, of the removal of a plaster cast from the lower limb or of venous thrombosis or is of the type known as angioneurotic, effleurage is usually indicated for its diminution or removal. A crepe bandage should be applied tightly at the end of each session and kept on until the next session. The massage should be given daily, sometimes more often. In the treatment of oedema due to heart failure, phlebitis, nephritis or lymphatic obstruction caused by carcinomatous invasion, massage is only a temporary palliative. The oedema about an infected area must not be treated by massage, and hereditary oedema of the leg (Milroy's disease) and oedema due to filaria (elephantiasis) are not benefited. The oedema that always occurs after an amputation, especially at the lower limb, should be treated not by massage but by continuous pressure bandaging, tightening several times a day.[2]

### Traumatic Periostitis

Since the periosteum is attached to a motionless structure—bone—the formation of adherent scars is harmless. Deep friction is, therefore, never required. The periosteum is painful because it is swollen, and no more need be done than to reduce the swelling by firm, but not painful, deep effleurage, given daily. If a subperiosteal haematoma is present, aspiration will much hasten the patient's recovery, since blood is absorbed very slowly thence.[3]

### Deep Friction

The most potent form of massage is deep friction. By this means alone, massage can reach structures far below the surface of the body. Since the source of pain in patients for whom manual methods are required so often lie in muscle, tendon or ligament, whether as the result of injury or repeated strain, a penetrating technique is clearly essential if such tissues are to be affected. . . .

When mobility is to be maintained at, or restored to, those moving parts which from their nature or position are apt to develop adhesions or scar-

---

[2]Cyriax & Russell (1977), p. 9.
[3]Cyriax & Russell (1977), p. 9.

ring, deep friction is often the method of choice, either alone (as in the case of tendons) or in association with passive movements (for some ligamentous lesions) or with active movement without tension or the healing breach (for minor muscular ruptures). An important part of the [operator's] knowledge consists in choosing and applying whichever type of therapeutic movement is best adapted to the patient's disorder.[4]

## Mode of Action of Deep Massage

A penetrating technique is required in the treatment by massage of deep-seated lesions. Given properly, deep friction has a dual effect. It induces (1) traumatic hyperaemia and (2) movement.

1. *Traumatic Hyperaemia* Enhancement of the blood supply diminishes pain. Apparently it acts by increasing the speed of destruction of Lewis's P-substance, the factor responsible for pain. Heat and counterirritants soothe for the duration of their application, also as the result of similar enhancement of blood flow. They have no lasting effect upon the type of lesion under discussion, because no other change than the circulatory is secured. Deep massage results in a more lasting hyperaemia and it appears to be in this way that the friction, though in itself painful, is found at the end of the session to have allayed the symptoms for a while. In other words, deep massage given to the lesion itself affords temporary analgesia, and during this period treatment can be given that pain would otherwise have prevented.

2. *Movement* By moving the painful structure to and fro, it is freed from adhesions both actually present and in the process of formation. Clearly massage applied parallel to the length of a structure follows the course of the blood and lymph vessels, whereas transverse friction does not. Hence longitudinal frictions merely move blood and lymph along, whereas *transverse friction moves the tissue itself*. In most conditions, there is nothing wrong with the circulation, hence there is no advantage in trying to alter it. I regard the lasting benefit that so often follows massage in muscular, tendinous and ligamentous lesions as accruing from the application of therapeutic movement to the affected part.[5]

## Deep Massage for Muscular Lesions

The main function of muscle is to contract. As it does it broadens. Hence full mobility in broadening out must be maintained or restored in muscles that have been the seat of inflammation, whether caused by one or by repeated strains. Resolution by fibrosis is occurring or has already occurred. The effect of deep transverse friction clearly consists in mobilizing the

---

[4]Cyriax & Russell (1977), p. 9.
[5]Cyriax & Russell (1977), pp. 10, 11.

muscle, i.e., separating the adhesions between individual muscle fibres that are restricting movement. If passive restoration of full mobility of a muscle is followed by adequate active use, these adhesions do not re-form; cure results.[6]

## Deep Massage for Ligamentous Lesions

*In recent cases*, after any oedema that may be present has been removed by effleurage, the site of the minor tear in the ligament should receive some minutes' friction. The purpose is to disperse blood clot or effusion here, to move the ligament to and fro over subjacent bone in imitation of its normal behavior (thus maintaining its mobility) and to numb it enough to facilitate movement afterwards. The least strength of friction which achieves these results is called for. Hence, when friction is started during the first day or two after a sprain, the ligaments need be moved only a few times. One minute's treatment thus suffices, since as yet there are no unwanted adhesions to break down. But it may well take ten to twenty minutes' effleurage and gentle friction to enable the patient to accept the one minute's valid treatment—actually moving the damaged tissue. When the lesion becomes less severe and tenderness is abating, friction maintained with increasing strength for five, ten, then fifteen minutes is called for.

When acute traumatic arthritis is present at a joint such as the knee, muscle spasm so limits movement at the joint that it is impossible to maintain the mobility of a ligament in the usual way, i.e., by moving the bones to and fro under it. In such a case the only ... alternative is to use the human finger to move the ligament to and fro over the bone in imitation of its normal behavior. This is the very mobilization that transverse friction achieves, provided that it is given deeply enough to reach the injured fibres of the ligament.

*In chronic cases* deep friction is given to fibrous structures such as ligaments in preparation for manipulation. The friction thins out the scar tissue by which the fibrous structure is held abnormally adherent, and so numbs it that rupture by forcing becomes tolerable. However, in the case of the dorsal ligaments at the wrist, the coronary ligaments at the knee and the femoral extent of the medial collateral ligament at the knee and the sacrococcygeal ligament, the massage is itself the mobilizing agent and no forcing of movement follows.[7]

## Deep Massage for Tendinous Lesions

In acute and chronic teno-synovitis the way deep massage acts is somewhat different. On logical grounds it has been widely held that teno-synovitis, being as a result of overuse, should not be treated by further friction.

---

[6]Cyriax & Russell (1977), p. 11.
[7]Cyriax & Russell (1977), p. 12.

Nevertheless this is the very condition in which massage achieves some of its quickest and most brilliant results.

The phenomenon of crepitus proves that roughening of the gliding surfaces occurs. The fact that slitting up the sheath of the tendon at open operation is immediately curative shows that it was the movement between the close-fitting sheath and the tendon that set up the pain. Hence it would appear that manual rolling of the tendon sheath to and fro against the tendon serves to smooth the gliding surfaces off again. While the causative overuse was longitudinal friction, the curative is transverse.

In those tendons that lack a sheath, deep massage acts by breaking up scar tissue at the insertion of the tendon into bone or within its substance. Since no sheath exists, there is no reason to suppose that some slight roughening of the surface of the tendon would cause symptoms. Deep friction provides the only method whereby the [operator] can bring lasting relief in these cases. The alternative is local infiltration with hydrocortisone, which disinflames the scar, but leaves this still in existence. Hydrocortisone, when it succeeds, is a quicker method of securing relief, but it is followed by a higher frequency of recurrence on account of the persistence of the scar.

Since the cause of teno-synovitis and tendinitis is overuse, no exercises follow. Splintage is quite unnecessary; the patient is merely told to avoid any exertion that hurts.[8]

## MASSAGE WITH CREAMS

When deep friction is given, the [operator's] finger and the patient's skin must move as one. The application of any cream, ointment or powder, or even previous heat leading to local sweating, makes the skin slippery and must be avoided. But for centuries laymen's expectations have been periodically aroused that rubbing in this or that cream or liniment has a curative value. The effect postulated is local, not systemic as in mercurial inunction for syphilis. Naturally, it makes not the slightest difference to the deeper tissues what is or is not rubbed into the skin; for all agents that penetrate are absorbed by the blood in the cutaneous capillary system and removed. Counterirritation results, of course, and the patient may feel a pleasant glow, but it is probable that, by drawing more of the available blood towards the skin, the flow through the underlying tissues becomes diminished for the time being. But minor ephemeral ischaemia is not likely to do good, since analgesic measures rely on an increase in the local circulation.

The usefulness of rubbing in any cream, liniment or embrocation, however convincingly advertised to the layman and, even more assiduously, to health professionals, is worth stressing. Thousands of pounds are wasted on these remedies by laymen and National Health Service alike. Such strik-

---

[8]Cyriax & Russell (1977), p. 13.

ing claims were made twenty years ago by Moss for a massage cream containing adrenaline that the Empire Rheumatism Council set up a subcommittee to investigate. It reported that whether adrenaline was present in the cream or not made no real difference to the result and that none of the systemic effects of adrenaline was noted.[9]

Those interested in Cyriax's techniques should consult the book, *Textbook of Orthopaedic Medicine.*

[9]Cyriax & Russell (1977), p. 14.

# 27

# Albert J. Hoffa

This discussion does not include a *complete* translation of Hoffa's text, for much of it would not be applicable today. However, a complete translation has been made, and the techniques described closely follow the literal translation.[1]

Hoffa uses what he describes as the anatomical method for the different parts of the body, following the larger vessels, and selecting specific muscles or muscle groups to be massaged in order. He states that the following general considerations should be kept in mind during massage. The force should not be rude or brutal; all manipulations should be gentle and light-handed so that the patient feels as little pain as possible. No point should be treated for too long. Hoffa's text does not advocate any massage for more than 15 min, even for a total body massage.[2]

No massage should be done through clothing. The part to be massaged should be as relaxed as possible. The joints should be kept in mid-position so that tension of capsule ligaments and tendons is at a minimum.

If the hands are rough, a lubricant should be used. Hoffa maintains that if the part to be massaged is covered with hair it should be shaved. The operator should start with the healthy part and massage gradually toward the injured area, always stroking with the venous flow.

---

[1]With the help of Ruth Friedlander, the author translated the first edition of Hoffa's book into English. Passages quoted in this chapter are from that translation, and page numbers refer to Hoffa's original text. Should the reader wish to refer to the most recent German text see Albert J. Hoffa. (1978). *Technik der massage* (14th ed.). Stuttgart, West Germany: Ferdinand Enke.

[2]Max Bohm. (1913). *Massage: Its principles and technic* trans. Elizabeth Gould. Philadelphia: Saunders. This book, which is representative of Hoffa's technique as interpreted by Bohm, states, however, that up to three quarters of an hour can be taken for massage of the whole body.

Effleurage should be used for beginning and ending the massage as well as between all other strokes. If the part is covered by thick heavy fascia, effleurage is not deep enough and greater pressure is needed. Therefore, the knuckles must be used. Pressure is not continuous, but swells up and down, starting lightly and becoming stronger, then decreasing again. The hand should not stick to the part but glide over it lightly. If the hands are moist, they should be washed with alcohol and rubbed with salicylic powder.

## HOFFA'S EFFLEURAGE TECHNIQUES

### Light and Deep Stroking

The following description of effleurage is applied to both light and deep stroking; the deep stroking differs only in the amount of pressure applied:

> The hand is applied as closely as possible to the part. It glides on it, distally to proximally. . . . With the broad part of the hand use the ball of the thumb and little fingers to stroke out the muscle masses, and at the same time, slide along at the edge of the muscle with finger tips to take care of all larger vessels; stroke upward (p. 2).

### Knuckling

Knuckling is a stroke particularly associated with the Hoffa techniques. In describing it, he says:

> If the part to be treated is covered by thick fascia, effleurage (as described above) is not deep enough. You need greater pressure, therefore the convex dorsal sides of the first interphalangeal joints must be used. Clench the fist in strong plantar flexion, knuckles in the peripheral end stroking upwards, gradually bringing the hand from plantar to dorsal flexion. Pressure is not continuous, swelling up and down, starting lightly and becoming stronger, then decreasing again. The hand must not adhere to the part, but should glide over it lightly. Knuckling should only be used where there is enough room for the hand to be applied (p. 2).

### Circular Effleurage

Hoffa often refers to what he calls *circular effleurage*. In regard to circular effleurage of the fingers he writes:

> To do circular effleurage of each single finger, stroke around each finger from its point to its base, with strokes that cover each other like the shingles of a roof. Execute these strokes with the tip of the index and middle finger of the right hand, held in opposition to each other, while you lay the volar surface on your own left hand underneath the fingers on which you are working to support them. To make this stroke more vigorous use the tips of your two thumbs (p. 51).

To adapt circular effleurage to the arm, he says, "Begin on the forearm, stroking around the joint and doing strokes in such a manner that they always end up in either the biceps or triceps group. While one hand supports, the other hand massages (p. 58)."

## Thumb Stroking

Hoffa uses an alternate thumb stroking on the foot. He describes its use on the dorsum of the foot by saying, "Massage each tendon sheath by means of strokes of the thumb, alternating from the base of the toes up over the ankle joint (p. 62)."

## Alternate-Hand Stroking

No description of alternate effleurage stroking could be found other than use of alternate *thumb* stroking on the foot.

## Others

Hoffa mentions the use of simultaneous stroking and the use of one-hand stroking, but does not describe the use of the one hand over the other for deeper pressure (pp. 29, 32).

## HOFFA'S PETRISSAGE TECHNIQUES

### One-Hand Petrissage

Place the hand around the part so that the muscle masses are caught between the fingers and thumb as in a pair of tongs. By lifting the muscle mass from the bone, "squeeze it out," progressing centripetally. On flat surfaces where this petrissage is not possible, Hoffa does a stroke using a flat hand instead of picking up the muscle. This type of kneading is recommended for use on small limbs (p. 9).

### Two-Hand Petrissage

Apply both hands obliquely to the direction of the muscle fibers. The thumbs are opposed to the rest of the fingers. This manipulation starts peripherally and proceeds centripetally, following the direction of the muscle fibers. The hand that goes first tries to pick the muscle from the bone, moving back and forth in a zigzag path. The hand that follows proceeds similarly, "gripping back and forth." This progressive movement is made easier by doing most of the work from the shoulder (pp. 9–10). On flat surfaces where this petrissage is not possible, Hoffa does the stroke using a *flat* hand, instead of picking up the muscle.

### Two-Finger Petrissage

Over parts where muscle bellies are flat rather than round, and one cannot grasp hold with a full hand (such as the back, or over places where muscles are overlaid by strong fascias) the most useful kind of petrissage is the two-finger petrissage. Grasp the part between thumb and forefinger. Press it out by making little circular movements from the shoulder, making the fingers move the skin along with the rest of the movement. Some people refer to this as "creepy crawl" or "creepy mouse," but neither term connotes relaxation. This author prefers Hoffa's terminology, two-finger petrissage.

## Friction

In describing friction Hoffa says:

> Put the thumb in the neighborhood of the part to be massaged, setting the index finger of the right hand on the skin of the part, more or less vertically. Penetrate into the depth, not by moving the points of the fingers on the skin, but by moving the skin under the fingers.
>
> In going deep, describe small flat ellipsoids with the point of the index finger. These follow each other as quickly and consecutively as possible. The finger joints and wrist are to be kept almost stiff and the elbow joint only makes small excursions. The main movement is made from the shoulder joint (pp. 11–12).

He uses the index finger of the left hand to intersperse effleurage with the friction strokes.

In reference to the use of other fingers or part of the hand for friction, Hoffa refers only to the thumb, using it either to fit better to some anatomical part or to rest the forefinger. He also suggests using both thumb and index finger to do friction at the same time.

Hoffa uses the *thumb, index finger,* or *both* for friction.

## Tapotement

In describing tapotement, Hoffa says:

> Both hands are held vertically above the part to be treated in a position that is midway between pronation and supination. Bringing them into supination, the abducted fingers are hit against the body with not too much force and with great speed and elasticity. Fingers and wrists remain as stiff as possible but the shoulder joint comes into play all the more actively (p. 14).

Hoffa used this hacking stroke routinely with all back massages.

## Vibration

Hoffa says that vibration may be done either with the points of the fingers or with the hand lying flat. The forearm is at right angles to the upper arm. The whole forearm is brought into a rhythmical trembling movement from the elbow joint, but the wrist and finger joints are kept as stiff as possible. Even though he describes the technique, he feels that it is better to use a mechanical vibrator (p. 15).

## Massage of the Upper Extremity

In describing stroking and petrissage of the limbs, Hoffa begins with the right forearm, dividing it into two groups, the flexors and the extensors. The patient sits facing the operator, with the arm in a neutral position between flexion and abduction, and the elbow at an obtuse angle with the radial side upward. The patient should be as relaxed as possible. Three or four times is enough of each stroke to accomplish the purpose of effleurage.

After stroking out the muscles, petrissage is given. As in effleurage the muscle groups should be kept strictly in mind. First, the extensors are kneaded, starting at the wrist and ending at the elbow. The hand lifts up the extensors between the thumb and the other four fingers, kneading them centripetally. Once having arrived at the elbow joint, intersperse a few effleurage strokes about three times before undertaking a kneading of the flexors in a similar manner.

The upper arm is divided into three muscle groups. Group one includes the biceps, brachialis and coracobrachialis; the second group is the triceps muscle alone; the third division is the deltoid, which is divided into two parts, the back and the front. Massage of the upper arm begins with the stroking and kneading of the biceps group. The triceps are then considered. One applies the hand to the back of the arm, beginning just below the olecranon, gliding upward in the external bicipital sulcus and then on to the outer edge of the deltoid and into the auxiliary pit. The posterior part of the deltoid is massaged before the anterior portion and the massage to the upper extremity is finished.

In massage of the hand, Hoffa does a circular effleurage of each of the fingers. In doing this, he strokes around each finger from its point to its base with strokes that cover each other like the shingles of a roof. He executes these strokes with the tip of the index and middle fingers of the right hand, held in opposition to each other, while he lays the volar surface of his own left hand underneath the fingers on which he is working to support them. These strokes he refers to as "shingle strokes (pp. 23–62)."

For petrissage of the fingers, he takes hold of the soft part from both sides between the thumb and forefinger of his two hands and picks them up off the bone (as best he can), while moving along the skin and describing small circles, squeezing and progressing from the point of one finger to the base of the other in a zigzag fashion. The rest of the hand is done with alternate thumb stroking from the metacarpophalangeal joint to the wrist, and knuckling is done to the palmar fascia. The massage of the foot is very similar (pp. 51–62).

## Massage of the Lower Extremity

Hoffa mentions turning the patient when treating both front and back of the lower extremity. (This technique is no longer widely practiced and it is felt that the patient should not be disturbed any more than is absolutely necessary.) Place the patient either on his back or prone and adapt all techniques so that anterior and posterior aspects of the lower extremity are treated from one position.

Hoffa shows an illustration of the patient seated, with his or her leg in the operator's lap (p. 23). This author doubts that were Hoffa alive today he would recommend a position where support of the limb is so poor.

For massage of the lower extremity, the patient is seated, with his or her leg in the operator's lap (p. 23). The hip is in inward rotation, the knee slightly bent for massage of the outer muscles, and the leg is rotated outward to reach the medial muscle groups.

Beginning with the lower leg, Hoffa divides the leg into four groups: first, the tibialis anticus with the extensors digitorum, communis longus, and hallucis longus; second, the peroneal muscles; third, the outer half of the calf muscles; fourth, the inner half of the calf muscles with the tibialis posticus, flexor hallucis longus and flexor digitorum communis longus. Taking the above named groups in order, they are effleuraged and petrissaged. On the first group, the usual effleurage is followed by a few strokes done with the knuckles, due to the strong crural fascia. Two-finger petrissage is also used on this group. At the knee joint, intersperse a few effleurage strokes and begin to knead again. The peroneal group is covered in like manner. The last two groups are massaged with the usual effleurage and one-hand petrissage.

Massage of the thigh is divided into the quadriceps; adductors; tensor fascia lata; biceps; semitendinosus and semimembranosus; and, the glutei. For massage of the quadriceps and adductor group the patient lies on his back, and for the tensor fascia lata he lies on his side. For the remaining parts, the patient lies on the stomach. All groups are given effleurage and petrissage in the prescribed manner, with knuckling over the tensor fascia lata. The glutei are divided into two groups, considering the oblique direction of the fibers that run from the trochanter toward the iliac crest and those from the greater trochanter toward the sacrum and then toward the iliac crest. The operator is seated on the side of the patient opposite the part being massaged. Both sections are given effleurage and petrissage.

## Massage of the Back

The back massage first considers the long, back muscles, with the stroke beginning at the limit between the back and neck. The stroke progresses downward, leaving the spinous processes free, with the tips of the first and second fingers performing most of the stroke (Fig. 27–1). As the hands reach the sacrum, they diverge laterally from each other and follow the course of the iliac crest to the inguinal region. There the stroke is ended and the upward stroke begins. The stroke returns in a similar fashion to the sacrum and proceeds upward to the hairline (Fig. 27–2) where the hands glide along the neck laterally to arrive at the sternoclavicular joint. After several repetitions of these strokes, knuckle effleurage follows to affect the deeper tissues. Two-finger petrissage is then given to the long muscles of the back.

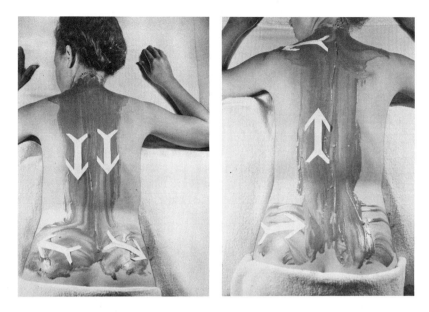

**Figure 27-1.** Erector spinae group.

**Figure 27-2.** Erector spinae group.

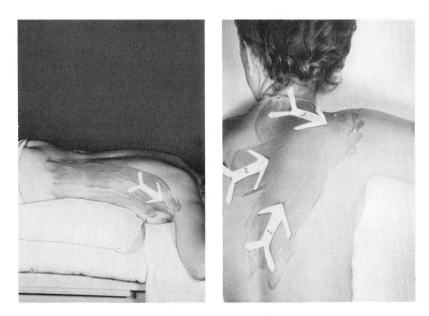

**Figure 27-3.** Latissimus dorsi.

**Figure 27-4.** Trapezius.

The fingerpaint patterns illustrate direction of the strokes and the area covered.

The latissimus dorsi is then effleuraged from origin to insertion (Fig. 27–3). The trapezius is divided into three groups in accordance with the three-fold fiber direction (Fig. 27–4). Each group is considered separately and given effleurage. This is contrary to the common opinion that Hoffa stroked the trapezius with an alternate effleurage stroke, but the description given here is upheld by Bohm.[3] Petrissage, using the flat hand, is given on the latissimus dorsi and lower and middle trapezius. Tapotement in the form of hacking is given after muscle groups have been effleuraged and petrissaged. All of one side of the back is done before moving to the opposite side of the table to massage the other side of the back.

## SUMMARY

The fact that Hoffa was one of the earliest to describe massage in a text, coupled with the accuracy of his descriptions, may account for the fact that his five fundamental strokes are still done today much as they were then, although the pattern or area of the stroke may vary greatly. These methods may still be used throughout America today, although those who use them are often unaware that they were written in German by Hoffa. It is hoped that this text will enlighten many and give Hoffa the credit that is most certainly due him.

---

[3]Bohm (1913), p. 73.

# ─28─

# Mary McMillan

Mary McMillan considered massage to be the manipulation of soft tissues or as movements done upon the body. She divided massage into five fundamental procedures: effleurage, petrissage, friction, tapotement, and vibration.

She believed that the student beginning to use the hands in various forms of manipulation had little difficulty in becoming accustomed to dry rubbing. McMillan prefered it, except in patients with excessive scar tissue, emaciated patients, or patients who wore splints for a long time. According to McMillan, cod liver oil or olive oil can be of nutritive value when absorbed through the pores of the skin, and would therefore be good lubricants to use if this type of nutrition is desired. Cocoa butter and lanolin are among the best lubricants, but should be used sparingly. The latter is preferred by some because it is an animal fat.

McMillan's massage was developed from her experience in teaching. Although it is not based on a particular method, she made reference to J. M. M. Lucas-Championnière, Sir William Bennett, Weir Mitchell, and Douglas Graham.[1]

McMillan maintains that one should first define the specific area to be massaged. For instance, in giving massage to the upper extremity begin from the fingertips to just beyond the wrist joint; second, from below the wrist joint to just beyond the elbow joint; and, third, from below the elbow joint to just beyond the shoulder joint.

It will be noticed in each subdivision that the stroke is carried from just below the distal joint to just beyond the proximal, the object being to carry

---

[1]Letter from Mary McMillan to the author, June 19, 1948.

the lymph to the proximal glands in order that it may be taken on through the lymphatics, back to the right side of the heart.

> An operator who cannot use one hand as well as the other is not only limited in performing the normal operations of the work, but is a 50 per cent worker. Therefore, from the start, one should practice more with the lesser developed hand as soon as some ability to perform certain manipulations is acquired. Great care should be taken to put pressure on the upward stroke, allowing the hand to return to its original position without pressure, but without losing contact with the part being massaged. The fingers of the operator in performing effleurage should be held close together, but not stiffly. Relaxation on the part of the patient is necessary. The greater the facility of the operator to mold the hand into the part being massaged, the better the work will be. This molding is making use to the utmost advantage of the span between the thumb and the fingers *en masse*. Most of the molding process is directed by the thumb and the thenar eminence. No jarring or jerking either at the start or finish of the stroke should ever be felt by the patient.[2]

Concerning treatment time and draping, McMillan says:

> There is no hard-and-fast rule, but the following table, stating the approximate length of time for the limbs and trunk, is given as an aid to beginners:

| | |
|---|---|
| Upper limbs | 10 minutes |
| Lower limbs | 15 minutes |
| Back | 7 minutes |
| Chest | 5 minutes |
| Abdomen | 5 minutes |

> . . . There is no need of exposing any part of the body other than that under treatment at the time. If there is any danger of the patient's taking cold, massage may be given under . . . a light-weight covering. If the patient wears a night-gown, each arm should be taken from the sleeve and replaced when treated. A light-weight but warm shawl is useful to cover the upper part of the back while the lower part is being massaged.[3]

## Joint Surfaces

Around joint surfaces pressure is brought to bear upon the underlying structures. In friction of the phalangeal joints the joints of the first and third fingers are manipulated between the finger and thumb of the operator. In the same way the second and fourth fingers receive friction. If friction is given simultaneously to alternate fingers, one hand of the operator is not in the way of the other. Friction is given around the wrist-joint with

---

[2]Mary McMillan. (1932). *Massage and therapeutic exercise* (3rd ed.). Philadelphia: Saunders, pp. 20–21.
[3]McMillan (1932), pp. 66–67.

two or three fingers and thumb. In the lower extremity the toes and ankle-joint receive similar treatment. In cases in which there is excessive scar tissue friction is the most useful form of manipulation to loosen it. . . .

Running frictions are sometimes used to advantage in a case of recovering sciatica. Over the denser area the thenar eminence is used for the circular frictions, starting over the great sciatic notch where the sciatic nerve emerges from the pelvis. These friction movements are carried down the whole area of the terminal endings of the sciatic nerve.[4]

## MCMILLAN'S EFFLEURAGE TECHNIQUES

### Light and Deep Effleurage

In effleurage, McMillan uses the whole of the palmar surface of the hand. Although light, the stroke is firm and even. The pressure is upward. The fingers are together and the hand is molded to the part. Most of this molding process is directed by the thumb and thenar eminence.[5]

### Alternate-Hand Stroking

Concerning alternate-hand stroking, McMillan says, "The third division of the lower extremity is the thigh. Here, because there is a larger surface to cover, it is well to stroke with alternate hands. . . . There should be about six alternate hand strokings over the posterior surface of the thigh. . . . "[6]

### Others

McMillan uses both *simultaneous stroking* and *one-hand stroking*, but does not make reference to the use of knuckling, thumb stroking, or one hand over the other for deeper pressure.[7]

## MCMILLAN'S PETRISSAGE TECHNIQUES

### One- or Two-Hand Petrissage

"Petrissage or kneading may be performed either with the whole of the palmar surface of the hand or by fingers and thumb."[8]

### Two-Finger Petrissage

"For picking up small muscles (as, for example, those of the face) the forefinger and thumb are used."[9]

---

[4]McMillan (1932), pp. 36–38.
[5]McMillan (1932), p. 19.
[6]McMillan (1932), p. 25.
[7]McMillan (1932), p. 24.
[8]McMillan (1932), p. 31.
[9]McMillan (1933), p. 31.

## Petrissage of the Back

For petrissage of the back, she says, "Each section in turn is petrissaged by a pressure of muscles against the ribs, or, in the lumbar region, upon the abdominal wall. These muscles cannot be picked up as those in the limbs. The whole of the palmar surface of the hand is brought into play, but not in a molding manner as for the limbs, because the contour of the surface is flat instead of rounded."[10]

## Alternate One-Hand Petrissage

"A useful variation of petrissage may be accomplished by the flexors and extensors being grasped by alternate hands, and a wringing movement being performed."[11]

## Friction

Regarding friction McMillan says:

> Friction, or circular friction, is that form of manipulation in which the tips of the fingers or the fingers and thumbs are used—more especially around the bony prominences of joint surfaces. Pressure in a circular manner is brought to bear upon the underlying structures. This form of manipulation is extremely useful in breaking down adhesions and in promoting absorption. Friction should be followed by effleurage in order to send on through the blood-stream the broken-down products of inflammation.
>
> Friction is performed by circular movements with the fingertips, or with two or three finger-tips, or even with one, according to the amount of surface to be coverd. . . . In friction of the phalangeal joints the joints of the first and third fingers are manipulated between the finger and thumb of the operator. In the same way the second and fourth fingers receive friction. . . .
>
> Running frictions are sometimes used to advantage in a case of recovering sciatica. Over the denser area the thenar eminence is used for the circular frictions, starting over the great sciatic notch where the sciatic nerve emerges from the pelvis. These friction movements are carried down the whole area of the terminal endings of the sciatic nerve.[12]

McMillan, then, uses the *thumb, two* or *three fingers*, or the *thenar eminence* for friction.

## Tapotement

> Tapotement is a series of brisk blows, one following another in rapid succession. It may be performed in four ways: hacking, clapping, tapping, and beating.

---

[10]McMillan (1932), pp. 33–34.
[11]McMillan (1932), p. 31.
[12]McMillan (1932), pp. 35–38.

Hacking is the most common form of tapotement. The operator's hands are held with ulnar borders of each ready to strike. The fingers are slightly flexed and parted, and the hands strike alternately. As the blow falls the fingers strike together. They are then separated, and the hand is raised some distance from the patient before the blow is repeated. Hacking is performed so as to strike transversely across the muscle-fibers from one end of the muscle to the other. . . .

Clapping is done with a cupped hand, the fingers and thumb being slightly flexed and the palmar surface contracted. This form of tapotement is especially useful for covering the entire surface of the back. Clapping is also used over the chest muscles. It has a stimulating effect when used over peripheral vessels and nerves.

Tapping is performed with the fingers cone-shaped, and sharp, brisk tapping movements are applied with the tips to the surface desired. . . .

Beating is done with the ulnar border of the closed hand, as in making a fist. This form of tapotement is used over the gluteal muscles where the fascia is dense.[13]

## Vibration

Vibration is performed with several fingers or even with one, and at times the whole palmar surface of the hand is used. A trembling sensation is conveyed by the operator. . . . [14]

## Massage of the Upper Extremity

In the first division of effleurage of the arm the palmar surface of the operator's hand supports the palmar surface of the patient's hand. The operator's working or active hand is then placed finger-tips to finger-tips with those of the patient; if the thumb-to-thumb method is adopted, it is much easier to fit hand to hand. Three or four firm, even strokings on the dorsal surface of the patient's hand are given. In order to conserve time and energy the operator, without changing hands, turns the patient's hand from the prone to the supine position; the supporting hand of the operator then becomes the active hand. The palmar surface is then stroked three or four times in a similar manner. In effleurage of the forearm the patient's hand is in the middle position between pronation and supination. One hand of the operator is used for the flexor group, while the other hand is supporting the part; then the hands should be reversed for the extensor group. The hands are now in position for effleurage of the upper arm, which is the third division. In a similar manner the flexor and extensor groups, each in turn, are stroked.[15]

McMillan then follows these same divisions, using petrissage and friction. She describes a useful variation of petrissage that may be used on

---

[13]McMillan (1932), pp. 38–40.
[14]McMillan (1932), p. 41.
[15]McMillan (1932), pp. 22–24.

both the flexors and the extensors. Grasping the flexors in one hand and the extensors in the other she performs an alternate wringing movement.[16]

## Massage of the Lower Extremity

In discussing massage of the lower extremity, McMillan states:

> Subdivisions of the lower extremity correspond to those of the upper: First, foot; second, leg; third, thigh. In effleurage of the lower extremity the same procedure is used as with the upper extremity. The leg which is being massaged should never hang from the knee-joint, but should be well supported from the hip-joint.
>
> The plantar surface of the foot from the tips of the toes to the heel is stroked with one hand. The other hand takes the stroke on the dorsal surface from the toes to beyond the ankle-joint. The whole palmar surface of the hand should conform to the sole of the foot.
>
> The leg should be grasped with one hand covering the muscles on one side of the crest of the tibia, the other hand grasping the muscles on the other side. In this way one hand covers the anterior tibial group and the peroneal, while the other hand grasps the gastrocnemius group, the underlying and posterior tibial group being affected by the pressure from the superficial group. Always, where there are several layers of muscles, especially where the muscles are much developed, the stroking should be deeper, in order to reach the veins and lymphatic vessels which lie nearest the bone.
>
> The third division of the lower extremity is the thigh. Here, because there is a larger surface to cover, it is well to stroke with alternate hands. At first both hands grasp the limb, finger-tips touching in the popliteal space, between inner and outer hamstring muscles. There should be about six alternate hand strokings over the posterior surface of the thigh, bringing the hands over the lateral aspects of the thigh to the anterior surface, where similar action is brought into play, until the whole of the thigh has been thoroughly stroked. This completes the general outline for effleurage of the limbs.[17]

McMillan then follows these same divisions using petrissage and friction. Concerning petrissage, she states:

> The lower extremity also is divided into three divisions. The foot is petrissaged, special attention being paid to the muscles of the plantar surface. The hand of the operator, making special use of the thenar eminence, kneads well into the plantar muscles. As the dorsum of the foot is so tendinous, petrissage is supplemented by running frictions between the interossei muscles. The spine of the tibia is used as a guide for the thumb of the operator in petrissage of the leg. On one side of the spine the muscles are kneaded by one hand, and on the other side of the spine by the other. If

---

[16]McMillan (1932), p. 31.
[17]McMillan (1932), pp. 24–26.

the small anterior tibial muscles require special care, finger-and-thumb petrissage is useful, as the muscle group is small and lies snugly against the tibia. In giving petrissage to the quadriceps group the two hands are used as one, the thumb of the right hand lying alongside the forefinger of the left hand, or vice versa. In this way the two hands, as one, pick up the anterior thigh muscles. The adductors and hamstrings are petrissaged by alternate hands.[18]

## Massage of the Back

It is well to divide the back into four main divisions, as there is so great an extent of surface. The patient should be in prone lying position on a straight plinth or bed with no pillows under the head. This position cannot be assumed by patients suffering from heart complication or from phthisis [tuberculosis] in which a hacking cough is aggravated by this position. In either of these cases, or when it is found inadvisable for the patient to lie flat, the back may be massaged while the patient is in a sitting posture. In general, however, the prone lying position is not at all uncomfortable for the majority of patients.

The first division of the back is from behind the ears, along the slope of the neck muscles, to the tip of the shoulder-girdle [Fig. 28–1 through 28–4]. At the beginning of the stroke the forefinger is separated from the other fingers in order to get well behind the ears, and the stroke is carried until all the fingers come in close contact with each other again at the nape of the neck. With the same firm, even pressure, the stroke is then carried to its termination at the acromion process. In this division both hands of the

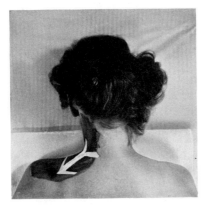

**Figure 28-1.** Upper trapezius, first division.

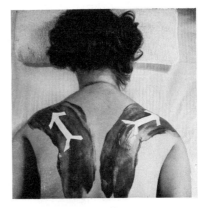

**Figure 28-2.** Middle and lower trapezius, second division. (Second division not discussed in McMillan's text.)

---

[18]McMillan (1932), pp. 32–33.

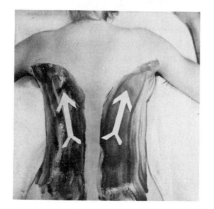

**Figure 28-3.** Latissimus
dorsi, third division.

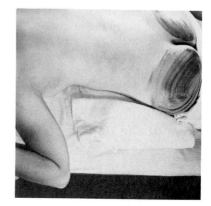

**Figure 28-4.** Gluteals,
fourth division.

operator start below the inferior angle of the scapulae and work in opposite directions from the center line, the stroke being repeated several
times.

In the third division the hands start over the region of the sacrum and
both hands stroke upward on corresponding sides until they reach the ax-
illa. They are then brought back, one on each side of the trunk, each describing a circular movement. Care should be taken to cover the whole
area with the upward stroke.

The glutei is the last division of the back. Here heavier pressure should
be exerted on account of the density of fascia in the region. The operator,
starting with one hand on each side of the buttocks, strokes from the apex
of the sacrum over the whole of the gluteal muscles, coming back without
pressure to the starting-point. When each division of the back has been
effleuraged, it is well to cover the whole surface with long, firm, even
strokes from the sacrum to the nape of the neck.

The back is divided in the same way for petrissage as for effleurage.
Each section in turn is petrissaged by a pressure of muscle against the
ribs, or, in the lumbar region, upon the abdominal wall. (sic) These muscles
cannot be picked up as those in the limbs. The whole of the palmar surface
of the hand is brought into play, but not in a molding manner as for the
limbs, because the contour of the surface is flat instead of rounded.

The glutei muscles and fascia, being dense, require a much deeper
kneading than those in any other region. The kneading movement over the
glutei is similar to that in kneading dough. . . . After effleurage, petrissage,
and tapotement of the first and second divisions of the back are completed,
those parts are covered to protect them. The third and fourth divisions
receive the same treatment, except that the glutei region, being more
dense, gets beating instead of hacking. The cover is now entirely removed
and the final procedure of effleurage is enacted, four to six strokes being
administered, and each stroke extending the whole distance from the sacrum to the acromion. Tapotement in the form of brisk tapping for its stim-

ulating effect, or light rhythmical hacking for its sedative effect, is used, according to the needs of the individual patient. Cupping the muscles, the hands being used alternately and making longitudinal sweeps each side of the spinal column, contributes the final procedure for the back.[19]

## SUMMARY

Mary McMillan's influence has spread throughout the United States, the Philippines, China, and Europe. Her dynamic personality carried her to far parts of the world, and wherever she went people could not help but feel her progressive influence. Through the army training schools, her techniques for positioning of the patient, maintaining contact on the return stroke, stroking off the whole area, and alternate-hand effleurage and petrissage became an integral part of massage in the United States.

---

[19]McMillan (1932), pp. 26–29, 33–34, 70.

# —29

# James B. Mennell

Mennell says very little about the exact technique of massage except to describe the various strokes. He classifies these as stroking, divided into superficial stroking and deep effleurage; and compression movements, divided into kneading, frictions, pressures, and petrissage. His terminology differs from common usage. He refers to friction as *frictions*, and divides petrissage into *kneading* and *petrissage*, the kneading referring to the circular, two-hand type of petrissage that is similar to McMillan's two-hand petrissage.

Most of the emphasis in his book is placed on a slow and even rhythm, a gentle and light pressure, and a longer term of instruction for the operator. A great deal of space is devoted to the physiologic effects accomplished by massage rather than on the actual technique. According to Mennell, it is of maximum importance in massaging a given part to begin away from the part which is injured or diseased and work gradually toward it.

In reference to the patient's relaxation, Mennell states:

> The resistance offered by muscular contraction in the part under treatment to deep stroking is so great as to render it practically useless. As the first essential is to ensure that the whole part is in a state of perfect relaxation, careful attention must be given to the posture, not only of the part under treatment, but of the patient's whole body. If necessary, relaxation must be procured by preliminary superficial stroking. If the muscles are relaxed, they offer to the movement no more resistance than so much fluid, and therefore it is obvious that any pressure, exerted on the surface, will be transmitted freely to all the structures under the hand. A pressure of 10 mm. of mercury will suffice to attain any objective desired by the use of the movement, except perhaps the mechanical emptying of a dilated lymphatic. A little practice, combined with a skill that is born only of a

delicate sense of touch, will show how very light may be the pressure which will suffice to compress any structure to its full extent, and therefore, incidentally, to empty the veins and lymphatic spaces. Also there is no call for great rapidity of movement. The flow of blood in the veins is slow, and of the lymph in its channels still slower. There is no object in performing a movement to empty a vein if sufficient time has not elapsed for blood to flow into it, since the last movement ceased. Moreover, a heavy pressure, a very rapid movement, or even a jarring contact may convey to the patient the fear of a possible chance of injury, be the fear conscious or subconscious. A protective reflex may then be excited, the muscle may contract, and so the one condition under which we can perform our work to the greatest advantage is sacrificed. . . .

Unless contra-indications exist, we may take it for granted that deep stroking should commence over the proximal segment of a limb before we attack the distal, so as to ensure the "removal of the cork from the bottle."[1]

Regarding the patient's position, Mennell points out that the patient should be generally comfortable, with the head supported, abdominal and thigh muscles relaxed, and the feet supported. The operator should maintain a stance which is, in general, comfortable, with no strain on the back muscles or knees. The position should be such that one can reach the whole limb and support it properly.

## MENNELL'S TECHNIQUES

### Superficial Stroking

Because superficial stroking is a distinctive part of Mennell's massage techniques, its description is included here in its entirety.

Though it is possible to trace a reflex response to most of the movements of massage, this is the only movement which aims at securing no other effect.

The essentials to remember in using this treatment are that our movements must be slow, gentle, and rhythmical and yet they must be given with what one can only describe as a confident touch; there must be no doubt, hesitancy or irregularity about it.

The slowness is important, as without it the other two essentials are impossible. If the stroke is to pass from hand to shoulder, some fifteen movements a minute will suffice. Moreover, the movement of the masseur's hand throughout must be continuous and even, not only while the hand is in contact with the part, but also during the return through the air, when there must be no contact. Occasionally we hear it stated that loss of contact between the hand and the part is conducive to a chilling of the

---

[1]James B. Mennell. (1945). *Physical treatment by movement, manipulation, and massage* (5th ed.). Philadelphia: Blakiston's Son; London: J. A. Churchill, pp. 28–29.

patient. This can only be due to inefficient performance, when the movement may convey a "creepy" sensation. This is usually the outcome of timidity, or of lack of training and practice.

The call for gentleness is obvious, as we are avowedly attempting to secure no mechanical effect. The firmness of the pressure should be sufficient only to ensure that the patient is actually conscious of the passage of the hand throughout the entire movement. Thus there should be no question of the patient being able to detect the passage of the hand over a certain point during one movement, while being unable to note it during subsequent movements. Otherwise the sensation conveyed by one movement cannot be identical with that conveyed by each subsequent movement. Firmness is essential, but only the lightest possible pressure.

The need for rhythm can be readily understood, as without it the nature of the stimulus will be uneven, and the reaction also will thereby be rendered uneven.

There should be no sensation of jarring at the beginning or end of the stroke, and the time that elapses between the end of one stroke and the commencement of the next must be identical throughout the whole of the treatment. To attain all these requisites it is essential to develop a "swing," and the portion of the "swing" which takes place while the hand is not in contact with the limb is as important as that during which hand and skin are in contact. Throughout the treatment the masseur's hand must remain supple, with all muscles relaxed, so that it may mould itself naturally to the contour of the limb, thus ensuring greater perfection of contact, and bringing as wide an area as possible under treatment. . . . If we wish to secure nothing but a reflex response to our movement, it may safely be left to the patient to decide the direction. If movement in one direction is more pleasing (i.e., more sedative) than another, there can be no objection to using it, even though the movement be centrifugal. Surface stroking "against the grain" of a hairy limb may be devoid of comfort, and, if so, it cannot be expected to call forth a beneficent reflex. It can only annoy. Shaving the part might be expected to help: it does not, and the process is not recommended save in the rarest of cases.

But whatever may be the direction chosen, one rule must be strictly obeyed, namely, that the stroking is performed in the one direction only. Thus, if we are stroking the back of a patient suffering from insomnia, our stroke should be from cervical or thoracic region downwards, or to the cervical or thoracic region upwards, never from sacrum to thoracic region and then out over the shoulder with a downward tendency at the end. In the same way, if a leg is being stroked upwards, the utmost care must be taken not to allow the hand to come into contact with any part of the limb during the return; otherwise the stimulus will be broken and the reaction thereby rendered imperfect. This is in direct opposition to the advice of a former writer to "feather your oars" when using stroking movements. By this he meant that heavy centripetal stroking should be followed by light centrifugal stroking. . . .

. . . The most common mistake is to scratch the patient with the pads of the fingers towards the end of each stroke. The second common error is to ignore the necessity for controlling the return of the hand through the air, and so to make this part of the movement less rhythmical than the stroking itself. A third main fault in technique is to ignore the necessity of selecting one definite direction for the movement, and, once having made the selection, of keeping to it. Another point, and one that is often over-looked, is that not only the hand, but every joint in the limb must be perfectly relaxed and perfectly supple.[2]

## Deep Effleurage

Mennell believes that this movement may be deep without being forcible, in any sense of the word. It is essential to ensure perfect relaxation (if necessary, this can be acquired through superficial stroking). A pressure of 10 mm of mercury will suffice to obtain any objective desired by the use of the movement, except perhaps the mechanical emptying of a dilated lymphatic. Since the flow of blood and lymph is slow, this stroke should not be rapidly executed.[3]

## Others

Aside from using *both hands simultaneously,* or *one hand at a time* as the occasion demands, Mennell does not use any other effleurage strokes.

Mennell distinguishes between kneading and petrissage; therefore, his description of both will be included here.

## Kneading

This is performed with the two hands placed on opposite sides of the limb, the whole of the palmar surface being in contact with the part. Gentle pressure is then exerted and a circular movement performed, the hands usually working in an opposite direction. Pressure is so regulated that it is not even throughout the movement, but should be greatest while the hand is engaged with the lowest part of the circumference of the circle, and least when at the opposite pole. This is effected by imparting a slight rotation to the wrist, the hand being more supinated below than above. The movement commences over the proximal portion of the limb; the pressure is then reapplied at the next most distal part and the movement repeated.[4]

## Petrissage

The movement consists of grasping the muscle-mass between the fingers and thumbs of both hands and raising it away from the subjacent tissues. The tissues grasped are then compressed alternately between the thumb of one hand and the fingers of the other. The hands are made to slide away gently over the surface, until the whole region has been manipulated. Care should be taken to avoid an all-too-common error in technique: dragging the fingers over the surface. Instead of merely exerting an intermittent pressure, the grip should be soft and the whole hand relaxed (Fig. 29–1). Occa-

---

[2]Mennell (1945), pp. 24–27.
[3]Mennell (1945), pp. 27–28.
[4]Mennell (1945), p. 31.

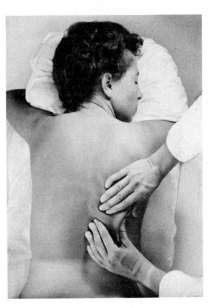

**Figure 29-1.** Mennell's petrissage to the back.

sionally, when the muscular tissue is sufficiently bulky, each picking-up movement is made to alternate with a kneading movement.

> A third method, applicable chiefly to the calf, is performed by picking up the muscle in one or both hands and carrying it from side to side with an inclination to upward movement at the same time. The result is an almost semicircular movement. . . . Any movement that calls forth a protective contraction can only defeat our aims, and should be regarded as an error in technique.[5]

## Friction

Regarding friction, Mennell says:

> In using frictions the object in view is to press deeply on the part under treatment and then to move the hand in a more or less circular direction. Any part of the hand may be used, but that generally employed is the tips of the fingers, or tip or ball of the thumb. . . .
>
> Friction directed transversely to the long axis of muscle fibers will often aid in securing relaxation.[6]

Although he says that any part of the hand may be used, he recommends the use of the tips of the fingers and the ball of the thumb.

Mennell's use of the term "frictions" instead of "friction" should be

---

[5]Mennell (1945), p. 39.
[6]Mennell (1945), pp. 33–34.

noted since he feels quite strongly that all massage is in a sense "friction," and therefore attempts to distinguish the terms by using this terminology.

## Tapotement

Mennell describes tapotement under the title of "percussion movements."

> *Hacking.* This may be performed with the ulnar border of the little finger, either alone or supplemented in turn by the other fingers—the result being a series of soft blows, the first from the little finger direct, the others from each successive finger in turn transmitted through the finger or fingers that have already delivered their tap. Sometimes the little finger is curled up in the palm of the hand, and only the middle fingers are used. If a more vigorous action is deemed necessary, the ulnar surface of the whole hand may be used with all the fingers kept close together and partially flexed but not rigid. The tips or palmar surfaces of the three middle fingers can be used. . . .
>
> *Clapping.* The hands are so held that the fingers and palm form a concave arch, and in this position they are brought sharply into contact with the body. The result is a rather deep-toned clapping sound. . . .
>
> *Beating.* This is the most vigorous form of percussion massage. The fist is half closed, and either the ulnar or the palmar surface is used for beating the surface of the body. If no force is put into the movement, it may be used over bony areas such as the sacrum and over areas well covered by muscle, such as the gluteal region. As our only hope from its use in these regions is to secure a reflex action it should be performed lightly.[7]

## Vibration

Regarding vibration Mennell says:

> Hand vibration is a poor substitute for many of the mechanical vibrators on the market. . . . It is true that a few—a very few—masseurs have been able to develop a technique of administering vibration with their hands to such a degree of proficiency that manual treatment is preferable to that derived from apparatus.[8]

## SUMMARY

Mennell's theory of "uncorking the bottle" by massaging the proximal aspect of the limb before the distal is now being practiced by most people. As a rule they are following his principle of adapting the treatment to the individual patient's needs, rather than treating by a specific routine which

---

[7]Mennell (1945), pp. 40–41.
[8]Mennell (1945), p. 44.

concerns the number of strokes or length of treatment given. His influence has been widely felt throughout the United States and Europe. His constant emphasis is on the gentle approach, beginning away from the sensitive part and working slowly toward it. His use of massage, combined with careful, relaxing, passive movement, is very effective.

# —30

# Body Therapies

The term *body therapies* covers a broad category of non-invasive techniques used by health care practitioners as enhancing tools, many of which involve massage. They can best be introduced simply by listing them. The author believes that all the following involve techniques already defined in previous chapters of this text. Many of them use one technique above the other, such as several methods of myofascial release that involve deep massage. These are combined with active and passive exercise and mental activities previously described and related to the patient's belief in the curing ability of the technique and the sincere intent of the therapist.

These therapies are

- Acupuncture.
- Rolfing.
- Postural ingratiation.
- Feldenkrais.
- ISPB (Integrated Psychophysical Balancing Technique).
- Hallerwork.
- Lami.
- Deep muscle therapy.
- Myotherapy.
- Neuromuscular release.
- Reiki.

The term *body work* is also often used. This term offends the author, who thinks of an automobile body shop rather than the caring exchange of energy involved in massage.

Brad Steiger writes about body therapy, Kahuna magic. He says, "If we modern people would combine Swedish massage, the various baths, chiropractic, osteopathy, the use of suggestion, and the ancient religious practice of the "laying on of hands," we should approach the scope of *lomiloma*, the ancient Hawaiian system of healing."[1]

## MANUAL LYMPHATIC DRAINAGE

As with other massage systems described in detail in this text, manual lymphatic drainage (MLD) should not be attempted without specific training by a qualified person. Even complete descriptions cannot teach that which must be demonstrated and practiced until the teacher is assured that the student is executing the technique properly. This is especially true with MLD, because unwanted side effects can result from improper sequencing. (For a schematic of the body's lymphatic system *see* Fig. 30–1.)

### Massage Technique

Vodder's[2] MLD could be regarded as one of the classical large-surface massage methods. To the casual observer, the manual techniques even resemble the antiplethoric manipulations of classical massage. A closer examination will, however, reveal that MLD is considerably more difficult as it involves manual techniques that are not used in any classical form of massage. All massage techniques have one thing in common: by contact with the skin they stimulate specific receptors, resulting in a specific reaction. The exact receptors that are stimulated and the effect this has depends on the manner of skin contact. The effect of MLD as described presupposes that this method is applied in its original form, as taught at the Vodder School in Walchee, Austria.

We can distinguish between four different techniques: stationary circles; pump technique; scoop technique; and rotary technique.

***Stationary Circles.*** The fingers are placed flatly on the skin and the skin is pushed either in the same place as "stationary circles" or as expanding spirals. These manipulations are used primarily for treating the neck, face, and lymph nodes. These stationary circles are varied on the body and extremities by making circles hand on hand or with eight fingers placed next to each other. In the latter case, the fingers can press the skin circularly in one direction working together or alternately. The direction of pressure is determined by the lymph drainage. The fingers lie flat—sometimes the whole hand does. Each of these circles is executed with a smooth increase of pressure into the tissue and a smooth decrease of pressure.

***Pump Technique.*** With this technique, the palms are facing downward. The thumb and fingers move together in the same direction, pressing the skin

[1]Brad Steiger. (1982). *Kahuna magic*. Rockport, MA: Para Research, p. 83.
[2]H. Wittinger & G. Wittinger. (1982). *Introduction to Dr. Vodder's manual lymphatic drainage: Vol. 1*. Heidelberg: Haug Publishers.

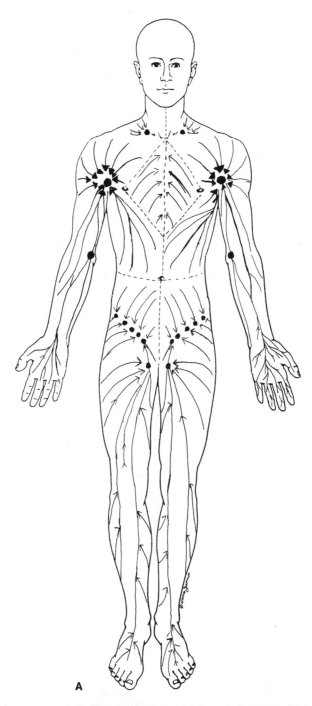

**Figure 30–1A.** Schematic representation of the body's lymph drainage of the skin (front view), with the collecting lymph nodes: "terminus," axillary lymph nodes, inguinal lymph nodes. (Vodder, E: *Die manuelle lymph drainage ad modum Vodder. Schema über lymphbahnen und lymphkasten.)*

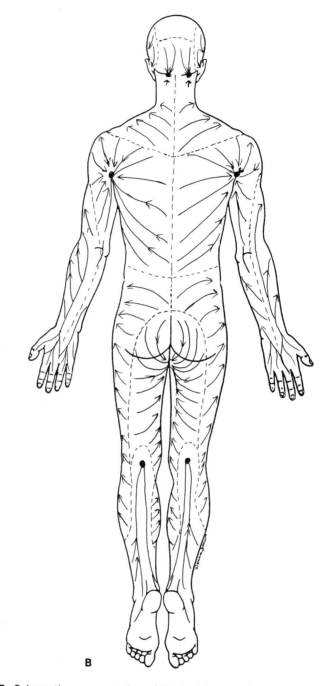

**B**

**Figure 30–1B.** Schematic representation of the body's superficial lymph drainage pathways (rear view) (Vodder, E: *Die manuelle lymph drainage ad modum Vodder. Schema über lymphbahnen und lymphkasten.*)

in oblong circles. This movement of thumb and fingers is controlled by the exaggerated movements of the wrist. The fingers are outstretched; the fingertips have no function in this technique. The wrist moves like a hinge. The forward motion of the fingers is carried out under pressure, the forward motion of the wrist without pressure.

***Scoop Technique.*** In contrast to the pump technique, the palm is facing upward. Vodder describes the movement as a "giving motion." The rotating wrist effects a corkscrew movement of the wrist–hand unit. The fingers are outstretched and swing towards the body during the pressure phase—with pressure in and without pressure out.

***Rotary Technique.*** This technique is used on relatively flat areas of the body and consists of various individual movements. The wrist moves up and down. As it moves downward, it swings from the outside towards the inside. The whole palm lies on the skin and presses it spirally inward. The thumb also makes circular movements in the direction of the lymph drainage of the skin. These motions are performed during the pressure phase. In the pressureless phase the wrist is raised, the four outstretched fingers keep on moving, and the thumb begins a new pressure cycle by completing the circular motion begun.

MLD consists of these four manual techniques, which may be combined in practice. It can be seen from the description that Vodder's MLD consists of a combination of round or oval, small or large, deep or shallow circular movements. The skin is kneaded, not stroked. For didactic reasons, this principle is handled generously in basic courses so that the direction of the movements becomes second nature to the student.

Precise execution of the manual techniques is then practiced in more advanced courses.

***Massage Dosage.*** The length of treatment of a particular body part, the use of certain pressure, and the speed of the movements can be explained, but not taught. Thus, the theoretical lessons are only an aid in explaining the effect of MLD and preparing the ground for an understanding of the value and use of MLD in physical therapy and health care. The dosage of MLD must, however, depend on the fingertip control and intuition of the therapist and cannot be taught, because in practice no two cases are identical. The description of MLD must be seen and understood with this borne in mind.

Since the effect of MLD is largely derived from the mechanical displacement of fluids and the substances they carry, it is essential that the manual techniques developed by Vodder be precisely executed. Experience shows that the more exact the technique, the better the results. The use of a certain pressure depends on the state of the tissue to be treated. One could say the softer the tissue, the softer the massage.

***Basic Principles.*** The following are a number of basic principles that are characteristic of MLD.

1. The proximal area is treated before the distal so that the proximal area is emptied to make room for the fluid flowing in from the distal end.
2. MLD prescribes a certain pressure intensity limited to 30–40 torr.
3. Each circular movement has a pressure intensity such that when the skin is released, the skin "snaps back." Think of moving *only* the skin with the pressure applied.
4. The direction of pressure depends on the efferent lymph vessels susceptible to the massage pressure.
5. The techniques and variations are repeated rhythmically, usually five to seven times, either at the same location in stationary circles or in expanding spirals. It is pointless to repeat the movements less frequently, because the inertial mass of the tissue fluid needs some time before it responds.
6. The pressure phase of a circle lasts longer than the relaxation phase.
7. As a rule, no reddening of the skin should appear.
8. MLD should not elicit pain.[3]

## SUMMARY

The two volumes of *Introduction to Dr. Vodder's Manual Lymphatic Drainage* provide excellent explanations of the autonomic pathways of the lymphatic system. As with the Bindegewebsmassage system, exactness of touch and location and directness of stroke are most important. Therefore, the overview presented is primarily to alert massage therapists to the value of this technique.

## THE TRAGER APPROACH

The Trager approach was developed by Milton Trager through 60 years of experience working with people of varying degrees of health, from the severely disabled to those who just wish to feel better. Coming from a varied background (he boxed in his youth, was an acrobat and dancer in his twenties, and then a doctor of physical medicine during World War II) Trager became a doctor of medicine in 1955 and practiced general medicine and physical rehabilitation for 18 years. Trager and his wife, Emily, have since dedicated their lives to the teaching and training of certified Practitioners of the Trager approach. Through his many years of work, Trager found the principle to be elegantly simple:

---

[3]Ingrid Kurz. (1982). *Introduction to Dr. Vodder's manual lymphatic drainage,* Vols I–II (2nd ed.). Heidelberg: Haug Publishers, p. 91.

We learn to love by being loved, we learn gentleness by being gentle, we learn to be graceful by experiencing the feeling of grace. . . . The goal of a Trager session is to bring to the surface of consciousness an awareness of this force of pleasurable and positive feelings.[4]

The Trager approach is not a technique or a method but, in a sense, an attitude—an approach to learning or relearning a way of allowing or enhancing movement reeducation that can bring more efficient use of our human body and mind. A Trager session consists of gentle rocking, and the movement of muscles, limbs, and joints to produce sensory experiences of light, freedom, and ease. The Practitioner uses his or her hands and mind to communicate this positive experience through the patient's tissue to the central nervous system. "When a body feels lighter it begins to stand and move as though it were lighter." It is an approach that can also reawaken the playful fun-loving child in each of us—allowing it to flow through the learning and wisdom of adulthood to merge into a new level of maturity that is filled with the delight at being alive.

The Practitioner works in a state of "hook up" as Trager calls it. This is a state of awareness that allows one to come into contact with that force or energy that is greater than any one of us. One can literally hook up to this something any moment one wishes and assist others to bring this awareness into their lives more of the time.

A lesson in "Mentastics" is included in each private session. Mentastics, a word the Tragers coined from mental gymnastics—mindfulness in motion—are profoundly simple dance-like movements that enhance or bring back this feeling of lightness, freedom, and flexibility. They are simple, playful movements that one can do at home to relieve accumulated stress and reawaken a feeling of lightness and aliveness. Mentastics are also offered in group classes and can be beneficial to people of all ages.

In 1975, the Trager Institute was founded to establish and support the professional standards for the Trager approach, and to train and certify Practitioners. Only those actually certified by the institute can use the Trager name and logo.[5]

## MYOFASCIAL RELEASE[6]

Myofascial release represents an important dimension in the health professional's evaluatory and treatment regime.

Fascia is a tough connective tissue that has an elastic component, a *col-*

---

[4]Dean Juhan. (September, 1984 through February, 1985). *The Trager approach: Psychophysical integration and mentastics.* The Esclan Catalogue, pp. 6–8.

[5]Personal consultation with Carolea Burgess. (1987). Written especially for this text. Used with permission.

[6]Written for this book by John F. Barnes, P.T. of MFR Treatment Seminars. (1987). Used with permission.

*lagenous* or plastic component and a matrix or ground substance that under normal conditions is a gelatinous-like substance. However, through trauma, inflammatory processes and poor posture over time, cross restrictions can occur within the fascia, and the viscosity of this ground substance can become solidified and shortened, ultimately pulling on pain sensitive areas that create symptoms of pain, etc. or restriction of motion. Fascia surrounds and infuses every system of the body all the way down to the cellular level. Fascia can create tensile forces of over 2000 lbs/sq in. when restricted.

The health sciences' failure to recognize the importance of a total physiologic system, the fascia system, is responsible for many of the poor or temporary results encountered. Meditation, biofeedback, physical therapy modalities, exercise flexibility programs, massage, muscle energy techniques, and joint mobilization and manipulation procedures address either the relationship between the osseous structures of the muscle or the elastic component of the fascia. Only myofascial release alters the *collagenous* aspect of the fascia and the viscosity of its ground substance.

Myofascial release is a hands-on technique that applies prolonged light pressure with specific directions into the fascia system. Myofascial release is not meant to replace the important techniques now presently being used by the various health professionals, but represents an important added dimension and is considered to be the missing piece of the puzzle for the health professional wishing to relieve pain and stress and restore function of the whole body.

### Janet Travell: Myofascial Pain and Dysfunction[7]

Travell has had success using Flurari Methane Spray combined with stretching. She has also used deep friction to release trigger points before stretching.

---

[7]Janet G. Travell & David G. Simons. (1983). *Myofascial pain and dysfunction: The trigger point manual.* Baltimore: Williams & Wilkins.

# PART V

# Supplemental Learning and Teaching Materials

# 31

## Cases for Analysis and Planning of Treatment Program

Regardless of the injury or illness of the patient, the operator will be dealing with such conditions as pain, swelling, scar tissue, muscle spasm, fibrositic nodules, muscle splinting, poor skin condition following casting, contractures, and insufficiencies of circulation. Students of massage should be exposed to other courses such as pathology, orthopedics, surgery, and neurology, in order to understand the injuries and illnesses with which they will be dealing. The following lists of indications and contraindications will give an overview of situations commonly treated by massage and those for which massage might do more harm than good.

### INDICATIONS AND CONTRAINDICATIONS

Each indication should be considered with the view that there are times when the patient might *not* profit by massage. No one can be expected to do an adequate job of massage without a thorough understanding of the medical implications of each situation. If a certain effect is desired, the operator must determine how it can be obtained.

In most of the following situations, massage would be indicated during a subacute phase *but not during an acute phase:*

- Cardiac decompensation.
- Edema, obstructive or decompensated, also inflammatory or noninfectious.
- Hematomas.
- Herniated disc.
- Mental states, particularly depressive or manic.

- Nonunion fractures.
- Phlebitis.
- Postoperative tendon transplants; orthopedic cases; neurologic cases.
- Severe lacerations.
- Spastic paralyses, such as Parkinson's, multiple sclerosis, hemiplegias, paraplegias, congenital cerebral palsies, traumatic or postsurgical brain injuries, encephalitis.

In many situations, the consequences of massage would be obvious to the operator, who understands its physiologic or mechanical effects. One must be aware of the damage that can be done by the indiscriminate use of massage.

*Any of the conditions listed under indications that appear acute should be considered as contraindicated for massage. In addition, one should be sure that none of the following conditions exists before proceeding with massage.*

- Pregnancy, large hernias, or any possibility of peritonitis or appendicitis are all situations where abdominal massage is contraindicated.
- Acute tubercular lesions, malignancies.
- Cellulitis.
- Certain neurotic conditions, especially emotional instabilities.
- Debilitating diseases.
- Edema due to heart decompensation or kidney ailments, synovitis, thrombus which may be dislodged, or embolism.
- Fever.
- Massage that aggravates the patient's mental or physical condition.
- Localized acute infections.
- Recent surgery.
- Skin eruptions that may exacerbate.
- Undiagnosed friends.

## CASES FOR ANALYSIS AND PLANNING OF TREATMENT PROGRAM

The following cases include the diagnosis and treatment prescribed. They have been designed for the purpose of helping students see the relationship between disabilities and the planning that is needed to organize the massage treatment. By thinking these cases through, one can relate theory and practice. Greater confidence will be developed, professional attitudes strengthened, and effective reasoning and problem-solving ability will improve. The organization of a case will increase understanding of the disorder.

Names, dates, record numbers, addresses, number and frequency of treatments, doctor's signatures, and dates for re-examination by the doctor have been deliberately ignored in writing the following cases. This is to focus attention on the massage. Such information is usually included in case reports, but here it would only be repetitive.

These cases include situations that involve many parts of the body and encompass conditions that are often treated by massage.

Users of this text who do not have adequate background or supplementary courses in anatomy, physiology, and pathology, or are not taking a course with a qualified instructor who can competently guide and correct their plans, will profit little by this approach and should not attempt to analyze these cases by themselves. *In some instances, these cases deliberately include situations that should not be massaged at all.* In these cases, students should know why massage would not be advisable. *In other cases, inadequate or inaccurate information is provided.* In such cases, the students should realize this and be able to state what questions need to be answered before treatment is given. *In several instances, the treatment ordered is incorrect.* In these cases students should seek accurate treatment instructions, or be ready to recommend more appropriate treatments.

The following outline will assist in the study of these cases. With the guidance and assistance of a qualified instructor, one can become more aware of the many things that have to be considered whenever a brief diagnosis is given. In each case, one should seek the following information:

1. Adequate description of the injury or illness.
2. Significant dates of onset, surgery, casts, etc.
3. Necessary supportive measures: braces, crutches, and support during treatment.
4. Treatment requested (is it adequate? accurate?).
5. Precautions, indications, and contraindications for the treatment requested.

In preparing to massage these cases one should consider:

1. Purposes of the treatment, such as reduction of swelling, increase in range of motion, reduction of pain, relaxation, etc.
2. Creation of relaxed environment, establishment of good social and professional relationship.
3. Additional information that might be needed.
4. Positioning and draping to be used.
5. Assistance with dressing and undressing.
6. Choice and use of lubricant, if any.
7. Organization of the massage treatment to include:
   a. Efficient use of time and equipment.
   b. Area to be treated.
   c. Direction, rhythm, and choice of treatment to be given.
   d. Pressure to be used, tolerance of patient to pressure.
   e. Body mechanics of the operator.
   f. Termination of treatment, equipment to replace, cleaning of treatment table, arrangements for next appointment, etc.
   g. Other types of treatment to be given in addition to massage.
8. Evaluation of effectiveness of treatment. (What observations can be

made that will indicate whether or not the objectives of treatment have been accomplished?)

## CASE STUDIES

Any of the previous situations can be used and written up according to the following outline.[1]

A. Case History (to include the following):
   1. Present date.
   2. Age and sex of patient.
   3. Diagnosis and pathology (also contributing factors or complications, if any).
   4. Significant dates (onset, surgery, casts, etc).
   5. Type of patient (wheel chair, crutches, ambulatory, etc; distinguish between hospitalized and out-patients).
B. Treatment ordered (mention all treatment ordered but elaborate only on massage).
   1. Type of treatment.
   2. Frequency of treatment.
C. Precautions.
D. Positioning.
   1. General position (sitting, lying supine, prone, etc).
   2. Support indicated (pillows, etc).
   3. Is elevation indicated?
E. Draping.
F. Type of lubrication.
G. Organization of routine (including amount of pressure used).
H. Duration of entire massage treatment (indicate approximately how time would be proportioned).
I. Termination.
J. Source of information for history and treatment.

## SAMPLE CASE

The following case has been analyzed for use as a sample.

### Information Provided for the Operator

*Diagnosis.* A 3-year-old boy has received a severe burn to the right wrist. There is extensive scar tissue and flexion contractures at the wrist joint.

---

[1]This outline was created by Vera Kaska, Instructor of Massage, University of Connecticut School of Physical Therapy. It is reproduced here with her permission.

*Treatment.* Massage to the right forearm and hand, in preparation for stretching.

## Analysis as Done by the Operator

*Description of Injury.* The description does not tell how the boy was burned nor when, nor how extensively the wrist is involved except that it was extensive enough to leave a scar and cause contractures at the wrist. Some of this information could be quickly learned by examining the patient. Usually, it is helpful to know how the accident happened. Such information could be obtained from the person requesting the treatment or the patient's chart.

*Significant Dates.* There is no indication of the date of the accident. This could probably be found by checking the patient's chart.

*Support.* No support should be needed other than for the comfort of the patient.

*Treatment Requested.* There is no request for heat preceding massage, nor for stretching of the contractures. One may suggest the importance of combining stretching with massage to regain normal motion. One should also initiate an exercise program.

*Precautions.* Be assured that the scar tissue is strong enough to permit this type of treatment and seek further information as to the extent of the depth of scar tissue. Review the pathology of burns.[2]

*Purpose of Treatment.* The purpose of massage in this case would be to promote relaxation, stretch tissue, encourage active motion, improve local blood supply, and increase range of motion.

*Gaining Confidence.* At the onset of treatment, gaining this little boy's confidence will be more important than the amount of motion regained. The approach should be friendly and gentle, causing no undue pain. When he is fully aware of the objectives of his treatment program he can then be asked to cooperate, even to the extent of enduring any necessary pain. Find out what he likes to do with his hands and encourage him to try to do all he can for himself.

## Additional Information Needed

One needs to know the depth of the burn, how it happened, whether the elbow flexors are also tight, whether the finger flexors are involved, and the condition of the scar tissue.

---

[2]Stanley L. Robbins, Ramze S. Cotran, & Vinay Kumar. (1984). *Pathologic basis for disease* (3rd ed.). Philadelphia: Saunders, p. 462.

## Position

Because the patient is 3-years old, he would probably be comfortable sitting on a treatment table with a pillow in his lap. This would put him high enough to work with easily. He might also be comfortable lying down on the treatment table, letting his arm rest on it.

## Draping

Remove his shirt. Leave the undershirt on if it has no sleeves. Put a towel about the shoulders.

## Assistance with Dressing

Let the parents help him until he is acquainted with the operator.

## Lubricant

Use cocoa butter, which has proven to be good for scar tissue.

## Organization of Treatment

*Time.* Allow time to become acquainted for the first treatment; possibly 30 min; later, massage could probably be done in about 15 min.

*Area to be Treated.* If the elbow is also tight from protective positioning, the entire arm should be included in the massage. The upper arm and elbow should be massaged before concentrated work on the wrist and hand is done.

*Choice of Technique.* Treatment of the upper extremity would be done as described in Chapter 14 of this text. In addition to this, deep effleurage strokes that stretch while they stroke should be carried out. By working into these strokes gradually, the patient will tolerate greater stretching. Stretching should never exceed the pain tolerance of the patient and should begin and end gradually. If there is no swelling, stretching strokes may pull downward against the venous flow. These should be followed by effleurage strokes that go with the venous flow. Keeping in mind that massage cannot break up deep adhesions or scar tissue, active motion should be encouraged. Much of the tightness present may be due to protective muscle splinting against pain. If this is so, good results can be expected. Treatment should be concluded with effleurage to the entire arm, working from deep pressure to light.

*Pressure.* Pressure should stay well within the pain tolerance of the patient.

*Body Mechanics of the Operator.* Body mechanics of the operator should be no problem with the patient on the treatment table.

***Termination of Treatment.*** Every effort should be made to finish treatment with the patient in good spirits and enthusiastic about returning for further treatment. Attention to the patient should take preference over clearing up the treatment area, which can be done when he has left.

***Other Types of Treatment.*** Although the prescription calls only for massage, combined stretching and active exercise should be included. This boy could also profit from occupational therapy to encourage functional reeducation for the entire arm and hand.

## How to Tell If Objectives Have Been Accomplished

If range of motion increases (determined by goniometer measurements compared with the first day of treatment), the major objective of treatment has been accomplished. If the boy relaxes and cooperates with the program, treatment will be more effective. If the functional use of the boy's arm continues to improve, it can be assumed that treatment is accomplishing the objectives for which it was designed. If no increase in range of motion is noticeable, he should be referred for other treatment approaches or to a different operator.

## SUMMARY

This is an example illustrating how cases may be analyzed and treated. Each person may think of different ways to deal with every case. Regardless of how it is done, the experience of working out programs for oneself is where the real value of this exercise lies.

## PRACTICE CASES

### CASE 1

**Diagnosis:** A 50-year-old woman has hypertension and is unable to sleep.

**Treatment:** Back and neck massage or total body massage to encourage relaxation.

### CASE 2

**Diagnosis:** A 20-year-old male's right shoulder and arm have just been removed from a cast after surgery to relieve recurrent shoulder dislocation.

**Treatment:** Give tapotement, effleurage, and petrissage to deltoid and trapezius in an attempt to increase circulation and relieve spasm.

### CASE 3

**Diagnosis:** A railroad worker lost his left foot when he fell beneath a train 6 weeks ago. Surgical repair has been done and a stump 7 in below the knee remains. There are flexion contractures at the knee.

**Treatment:** Give massage to the left leg, including gentle to increasing percussion to the stump end.

### CASE 4

**Diagnosis:** A 55-year-old taxi driver has had severe bursitis in the right shoulder for 2 years.

**Treatment:** Give heat, massage, and exercise to the right shoulder.

### CASE 5

**Diagnosis:** A football player suffered a torn semilunar cartilage in the previous week's game. The knee is swollen and tender. He cannot bear weight on it.

**Treatment:** Very light massage to reduce spasm and pain.

### CASE 6

**Diagnosis:** A 43-year-old woman suffered amputation of the left breast 2 weeks ago due to a malignant tumor. The shoulder is painful and motion is limited.

**Treatment:** Massage to relieve pain and increase motion.

### CASE 7

**Diagnosis:** A truck driver crushed his foot, receiving multiple fractures, 8 weeks ago. The foot is swollen and painful. Motion at the ankle joint is limited. Recent x-rays show all fractures have healed.

**Treatment:** Massage to reduce swelling and pain, and to increase motion of all joints involved. Preheat the part by using whirlpool at 110° F and follow massage with exercise.

### CASE 8

**Diagnosis:** A paraplegic woman has developed a large decubitus ulcer over the sacrum.

**Treatment:** Massage surrounding tissues to stimulate circulation.

### CASE 9

**Diagnosis:** A 15-year-old girl was in an automobile accident. She has a fractured right femur that confines her to bed, in traction. In addition to the femur, there are fractures to the jaw and left elbow. She complains of severe pain in the back due to the uncomfortable position caused by traction to the leg.

**Treatment:** Give massage to the back. Move this patient as little as possible.

### CASE 10

**Diagnosis:** Onset of polio was diagnosed ten days ago in a 10-year-old boy. He has severe spasm of the hamstrings of both legs.

**Treatment:** Hot pack and massage both lower extremities.

## CASE 11

**Diagnosis:** A 40-year-old professor has severe low back pain from a herniated disc with severe sciatica associated. Any right leg movements stretching the sciatic nerve are painful.

**Treatment:** Give petrissage to the low back.

## CASE 12

**Diagnosis:** A boy received a greenstick fracture of the right ulna 2 weeks ago. The cast was removed two days ago.

**Treatment:** Give massage to the right arm.

## CASE 13

**Diagnosis:** A patient was operated on for a herniated disc at the fourth cervical level 1 week ago. There is slight swelling in the area.

**Treatment:** Massage, attempting to reduce swelling and relieve associated muscle spasm.

## CASE 14

**Diagnosis:** A 35-year-old woman received a fracture of the right humerus 6 weeks ago. The cast has been removed. There is limitation of motion at the shoulder and the elbow. The skin is irritated and tender. Heat has been applied.

**Treatment:** Massage in preparation for passive motion of the arm and shoulder.

## CASE 15

**Diagnosis:** A 43-year-old woman has a suspected tumor at the C-3 level.

**Treatment:** Give deep massage, both petrissage and tapotement.

## CASE 16

**Diagnosis:** A 45-year-old laborer suffers with myositis of the right upper trapezius.

**Treatment:** Give heat and massage to relieve pain and relax spasm.

## CASE 17

**Diagnosis:** A neuropsychiatric patient is 25 years old and in a maniac depressive state.

**Treatment:** Give back massage for sedation.

## CASE 18

**Diagnosis:** A patient has had severe arthritis of the whole body for the past 15 years. There is marked limitation of motion in the left knee; no motion of the patella; and a flexion of deformity of the knee at 145°.

**Treatment:** Give massage to mobilize the left knee.

## CASE 19

**Diagnosis:** The cast has just been removed from a well-healed fracture of the right elbow of an 8-year-old boy.

**Treatment:** Massage and exercise to mobilize the joint and strengthen the muscles.

## CASE 20

**Diagnosis:** A female, aged 57, fell and dislocated her left shoulder 4 weeks ago. She carries her arm in a splint. There is also a stretch injury to the brachial plexus.

**Treatment:** Massage the entire shoulder, arm, and hand, being careful not to change the position of the shoulder.

## CASE 21

**Diagnosis:** A 30-year-old concert pianist suffers from chronic tenosynovitis of the middle finger of the left hand.

**Treatment:** Give paraffin bath to be followed by massage.

## CASE 22

**Diagnosis:** A college basketball player sprained his ankle yesterday. There is considerable swelling; much pain exists.

**Treatment:** Massage in attempt to decrease swelling and get this player back into the game as soon as possible.

## CASE 23

**Diagnosis:** A boy's elbow was hyperextended when he fell while ice skating, causing some tearing of the ligaments. Extension to 150° elicits pain. There is slight swelling and discoloration; the elbow is still tender.

**Treatment:** Heat has been applied. Massage in an attempt to reduce swelling and alleviate pain.

## CASE 24

**Diagnosis:** A young female patient has had acute myositis of the left tibialis anterior since an automobile accident about a year ago. There remains an area of "hardness" in the midshin region that limits the contracting range of the muscle.

**Treatment:** Massage to increase range of motion of the ankle joint.

## CASE 25

**Diagnosis:** A 50-year-old bricklayer has chronic low back pain from an old lumbosacral strain.

**Treatment:** Massage.

## CASE 26

**Diagnosis:** A 50-year-old man has Bell's palsy on the right side following surgery for removal of a nonmalignant tumor of the parotid gland.

**Treatment:** Massage.

## CASE 27

**Diagnosis:** A professor has been having tension headaches involving spasm of the muscles of the upper back and neck, especially on the right side.

**Treatment:** Massage to relieve tension in upper back and neck.

## CASE 28

**Diagnosis:** An 18-year-old boy has a "baseball finger," the index finger of the right hand with a chip fracture of the metacarpophalangeal joint. There is pain and swelling.

**Treatment:** Give heat, massage, and active exercise.

## CASE 29

**Diagnosis:** A gunshot wound was received when a 30-year-old man was cleaning his rifle. A .22 caliber bullet entered his body just below the right clavicle and emerged through the right scapula, shattering that bone and piercing the brachial plexus. The patient was injured 6 months ago and there has been no return of innervation from the damaged peripheral nerves. He carries his arm close to his body in a sling and complains of pain throughout the entire shoulder and arm.

**Treatment:** Give heat, and massage prior to faradic muscle testing.

## CASE 30

**Diagnosis:** A 25-year-old butcher cut his arm just below the right elbow. The ulnar nerve injury had surgical repair weeks ago.

**Treatment:** Give massage to the right lower arm and hand to increase circulation. Caution! Do not extend the elbow.

## CASE 31

**Diagnosis:** A 60-year-old man has had arthritis of the spine. He stands in a slightly flexed position. Extension to normal standing position produces pain.

**Treatment:** Heat and massage to relieve pain and spasm.

## CASE 32

**Diagnosis:** A 25-year-old secretary has a cervical rib causing peripheral neuritis of the right upper extremity.

**Treatment:** Massage to relieve pain.

### CASE 33

**Diagnosis:** A 16-year-old girl has a fracture of the neck of the right humerus following an automobile accident. She has been out of the cast for two days. There is little range of motion of the shoulder, elbow, wrist, or hand. There is swelling and pain.

**Treatment:** Massage in preparation for mobilization.

### CASE 34

**Diagnosis:** A normal 20-year-old male is a star member of his college football team. Whether his team can win tomorrow will depend a great deal on how fast he can run and how far he can kick.

**Treatment:** Massage to precondition the player for peak performance the following day.

### CASE 35

**Diagnosis:** Casting has just been removed from a 4-year-old girl to correct bilaterally, congenitally dislocated hips.

**Treatment:** Use whirlpool followed by massage.

### CASE 36

**Diagnosis:** A 10-year-old girl fell on the way home from the grocery store, breaking a bottle of milk and severely cutting the thenar eminence of her right hand on the broken fragments of glass. Tendon repair was done ten days ago.

**Treatment:** Very cautiously massage, preceding with heat, and following with gentle active exercise.

### CASE 37

**Diagnosis:** A computer programmer has developed a severe subdeltoid bursitis that inhibits her capacity to work.

**Treatment:** Use ultrasound, massage, and exercise.

### CASE 38

**Diagnosis:** A woman slipped going downstairs into the subway station, fracturing the posterior aspect of the right calcaneus, 4 weeks ago. She is suing the subway for injuries received, which may be the factor accounting for her seeming reluctance to regain normal range of motion.

**Treatment:** Give massage and exercise.

### CASE 39

**Diagnosis:** A young woman fell from a horse 3 weeks ago. She was wearing glasses with metal frames. As she was dragged, with one foot caught in the stirrup, her face was deeply cut, tearing it from the lateral aspect of the right eye toward the mouth. The formation of keloid causes more disfiguration than normal and some adhesions are beginning to develop.

**Treatment:** Massage to loosen peripheral, adhesive scar tissue. If keloid formation increases refer her to a plastic surgeon for further treatment.

## CASE 40

**Diagnosis:** A patient is just recovering from surgical treatment for Carpal Tunnel syndrome. The right hand is weak and painful. The finger flexors are tight, and the patient seems reluctant to try using his hand for daily activities.

**Treatment:** Give heat, massage, and exercise to assist the patient in regaining use of the hand.

## CASE 41

**Diagnosis:** A patient has hysterical paralysis of both lower extremities following real, but nonparalytic polio. His younger sister suffers from paralysis of both lower extremities following polio just previous to the onset of her brother's.

**Treatment:** Give heat, massage, and exercise to support psychotherapy. This patient is to be approached exactly as if his paralysis were real. Any sign of muscle reeducation should be enthusiastically encouraged.

## CASE 42

**Diagnosis:** A 21-year-old man had a triple arthrodesis 4 weeks ago for correction of a club foot.

**Treatment:** Massage in preparation for mobilization of foot.

## CASE 43

**Diagnosis:** An 85-year-old woman had a total replacement of the right hip 1 week ago following a nonunion fracture of the head of the femur.

**Treatment:** Give heat, massage, and exercise to the right hip.

## CASE 44

**Diagnosis:** All fingers of the left hand of a 27-year-old woman were crushed in the car door of the family station wagon. There were multiple fractures of all fingers across the tips, with some chip fractures into the first joint. The nail of the middle finger is off and those of the others in various stages of recovery.

**Treatment:** Massage the left hand, especially the fingers, in preparation for exercise to regain normal function of the hand.

## SUMMARY

No one student can do justice in analysis of all these cases. Some can be assigned, whereas others can be used for group discussion. Others can be used in laboratory practice sessions. Any use made of them will increase the ability of people to meet and solve problems similar to those they will soon be facing. Any or all the techniques discussed in this text should be considered when planning a treatment program.

# Review Questions

**These questions are designed to help people who wish to review this material for qualifying examinations.**

1. Define massage.

2. On what basis would you judge treatment time for various patients?

3. Outline the important factors of the operator's personal appearance and cleanliness.

4. What postural considerations are important to the operator?

5. Name ten ways to assure comfort for the patient.

6. Name four fundamental facts pertaining to proper positioning of patients.

7. Outline the basic principles for draping a patient.

8. List the deciding factors in choice of lubricant or the use of none.

9. Name six lubricants and tell when you might use each.

10. Describe effleurage.

11. Diagram draping and positioning for massage of the back.

12. When the patient is lying prone, what consideration should be given to the position of the arms?

13. Describe all variations of effleurage.

14. Define the usefulness of petrissage.

15. List ten desirable qualities of personality of the operator.

16. Describe draping of the lower extremity, face-lying.

17. Briefly explain the place each name has in the history of massage and rearrange the names chronologically.

| | |
|---|---|
| a. Ambroise Paré | n. Sir William Bennett |
| b. Harving Nissen | o. Janet Travell |
| c. Albert Hoffa | p. Ruth Rice |
| d. J. M. M. Lucas-Championnière | q. Steve Kitts |
| e. Mary McMillan | r. Jasmine Wolf |
| f. Hwang Ti | s. Pauline Sasaki |
| g. Hippocrates | t. Milton Trager |
| h. Per Henrik Ling | u. Jack Meager |
| i. Gertrude Beard | v. Dolores Krieger |
| j. Homer | w. Frances Tappan |
| k. Siegel | x. Gertrude Beard |
| l. James B. Mennell | y. James Cyriax |
| m. Elisabeth Dicke | |

18. How can you judge how much lubricant to use?

19. How does Storms' technique vary from the usual type of friction?

20. Would you ever give massage for skin nutrition only?

21. What is the effect of massage on sensory nerve endings?

22. How would you know when it is safe to massage scar tissue following burns?

23. What would massage do to affect normal function of the skin?

24. What is meant by reflex effects?

25. List the mechanical effects of massage.

26. Why should massage be done slowly if the objective is to assist the lymphatic flow?

27. Why is it important to rid the muscle of stagnant by-products of fatigue?

28. Explain how muscles normally maintain a metabolic balance.

29. Why is massage useful following overactivity?

30. Describe the metabolic picture following underactivity.

31. What is meant by venostasis?

32. Name three instances when you would *not* massage situations showing venostasis.

33. Name and explain four causes of edema.

34. Why does swelling occur in dependent limbs when normal activity has been limited?

35. Will massage be useful in eliminating edema in limbs suffering from extreme activity?

36. Why is massage not recommended in cases where edema is the result of recent injury?

37. Why is research in massage so difficult?

38. Will massage reduce obesity?

39. Of what use is massage following peripheral nerve injuries?

40. Does massage affect total blood flow?

41. Is massage more effective than electrical stimulation or passive exercise in increasing the flow of lymph?

42. Can massage ever adequately substitute for active exercise?

43. Describe massage as done by Cyriax.

44. Name five of the most used acupuncture points and list disabilities which could be relieved by finger pressure at these points, or combinations of these points.

45. Differentiate between Shiatsu and Oriental massage.

46. Discuss the possible mechanisms for relief of pain by massage or therapeutic touch.

47. List five areas on the foot where finger pressure (reflexology) could relieve symptoms in specific areas of the human body.

48. Discuss the importance of concern and empathy for a person while giving any kind of treatment that involves touching.

# Summary Chart of Comparative Techniques

The following summary chart shows the results of a questionnaire done by the author in 1948 determining the amount of use generally given to the various massage techniques. Twenty-five graduate operators were interviewed from 15 different schools. These schools were: D.T. Watson School of Physical Therapy (Leetsdale, Penn); Children's Hospital (Los Angeles); Harvard University, Medical School, Courses for Graduates (Boston); University of Southern California (Los Angeles); Mayo Clinic (Rochester, Minn); University of Minnesota (Minneapolis); Northwestern University, Medical School (Chicago); New York University, School of Education (New York City); Stanford University (Stanford, Calif); University of Wisconsin, Medical School (Madison, Wis); Reed College* (Portland, Ore); Fitzsimmons General Hospital* (Denver); O'Reilly General Hospital* (Springfield, Mo); Walter Reed General Hospital* (Washington, D.C.); and The Institute of Southern Sweden (Stockholm).

In order to prevent any one school from influencing the results, not more than three from each school were interviewed. In some instances, when the operator was teaching in one school but a graduate of another, the information gathered was considered representative of the school in which that person was currently teaching.

---

*Army training schools.

**TABLE 1-1. SUMMARY CHART OF COMPARATIVE TECHNIQUES**[a]

| Question | Hoffa | McMillan | Mennell | Conclusions from Questionnaire Results |
|---|---|---|---|---|
| 1. Are there any exceptions to following the venous flow? | The only exception is in the massage of the back, where the stroke may go in either direction | No exceptions are made | Exceptions include superficial stroking and following the principle of beginning away from the injured area | The trend seems to be progressively toward making exceptions to following the venous flow as Mennell does |
| 2. What do you consider adequate treatment time for the back, a limb, and total body? | 6 to 10 min is used for back or limb and 15 min for whole body | 10 to 15 min is recommended for beginners to use for the back or limb and not more than 50 minutes for a general massage | Treatment time must depend on the pathology and reaction of the patient. No time can be suggested | Treatment time must be adjustable to the pathology and reactions of the patient, but average between 10 to 20 min for back or limb and up to 45 for the whole body, which is more than Hoffa recommends and similar to McMillan's suggested time |
| 3. What do you prefer as a medium? | Anything to make the part pliable can be used | Dry rubbing is preferred but for certain pathologies oil, cocoa butter, or lanolin is suggested | Mennell's prescription combines oil of Bergamot and French chalk | Except in cases where pathology demands one or the other, choice of medium is up to the therapist, as Hoffa suggests |
| 4. Do you massage by muscle groups or is massage done by other anatomical divisions of the body? | All massage is done by dividing the body into various muscle groups | Some areas are divided by muscle groups and others, such as the back, are divided using other anatomical landmarks | Only the fact that one begins away from the injured part and works toward it, is mentioned as to how the area is covered | The majority of operators still divide the body into specific muscle groups for massage as Hoffa does |
| 5. Is the most proximal part of the limb massaged before the distal? | Every description of a part to be massaged progresses from the distal aspect of the limb to the proximal | Descriptions progress from the distal aspect of the limb to the proximal | The proximal aspect of a limb should always be massaged before the more distal | The practice of massaging the most proximal aspect of a limb before the distal as Mennell recommends is now being widely used |
| 6. Is the whole extremity or back effleuraged before petrissage is begun? | Each muscle or muscle group is given effleurage and petrissage before the next group is begun | Massage of the leg is done by giving effleurage to the whole lower leg and then petrissage | No definite routine in this respect is stated | Most operators are still following the technique of massaging each muscle or muscle group with effleurage and petrissage before going to the next group as Hoffa does, rather |

|  | | | | |
|---|---|---|---|---|
| | | | | than effleuraging a whole part and then giving it petrissage |
| 7. Is the patient always placed in a recumbent position? | The only time that the patient is in a recumbent position is in massage of the back, and even here the patient may be in a seated position | The patient is always in a recumbent position unless pathology is such that this position cannot be held comfortably | The patient is preferred in a recumbent position, but each patient must be considered individually. Thus sitting, or even standing, positions may be used if necessary | Most massage to the upper extremity is done with the patient in a seated position. The tendency seems to be that of making exceptions to the recumbent position as Mennell does |
| 8. Which parts are usually supported, (1) in a back-lying position; and (2) in a face-lying position? | (1) No back-lying position is described; (2) No mention of support is made with reference to the face-lying position | (1) A rolled towel is placed under the knee; (2) A small pillow is placed under the abdomen | (1) Support is placed under the knee; (2) The body is supported in slight hyperextension for back massage, with one pillow under the legs and another under the chest | (1) Knees are supported in the back-lying position as by McMillan and Mennell; (2) Most people follow the technique of McMillan and support the abdomen, and all but three support the ankles or have them over the edge of the plinth |
| 9. What arm position is preferred when the patient is face-lying? | The arms are "out horizontally" | Arms are shown in T position and also down at the sides | Arms are folded over the head (chest is supported by a pillow which relieves weight on the arms) | McMillan's two positions are the ones used the most (T and at the sides), but the patient's comfort and ability to relax is the primary guide for selection of arm position |
| 10. In massage of the lower extremity is the patient usually turned from back-lying to face-lying? | The patient is turned to make the posterior thigh more accessible and is placed on the side to massage the tensor fascia lata | The patient is not usually turned, but may be if pathologic conditions are such that it seems best to do so | The patient is turned to make the posterior thigh more accessible | McMillan's policy of not turning the patient unless pathology indicates its necessity seems to be followed |
| 11. Must the part being massaged always be in elevation? | Hoffa seems to prefer a neutral position | All illustrations show the part in a neutral position | Elevation is preferred whenever possible | Following Hoffa and McMillan, the trend is still that of elevating the part for pathologic conditions and treating it otherwise in a neutral position |

*(cont.)*

323

**TABLE 1-1.** *(Continued)*

| Question | Hoffa | McMillan | Mennell | Conclusions from Questionnaire Results |
|---|---|---|---|---|
| 12. Is emphasis placed on stance of the therapist? | No reference is made to stance | No reference is made to stance | Mennell mentions the operator should stand at the side of the table and not at the end. One should be comfortable, with no strain on the back or knees | Little emphasis other than good body mechanics is placed on stance by everyone |
| 13. Do you alternate sides of the table during massage of the back? | The operator is instructed to move to the opposite side of the back when doing the other side | No reference is made as to alternating sides of the table in massage of the back | Mennell does alternate sides of the table during a back massage | McMillan and the majority of the operators do not alternate sides of the table during massage of the back |
| 14. Do you always massage in a standing position? | Most of the massage is done with the operator seated, even in giving a massage to the back | All illustrations show the operator in a standing position | It is advised that all massage be done in a standing position | Whereas people do not remain seated to the extent that Hoffa did, neither do they stand without exception. Hands and forearms are usually done with the operator seated |

| Question | Hoffa | McMillan | Mennell | Conclusions |
|---|---|---|---|---|
| 15. Do you usually repeat a given stroke any particular number of times before progressing to a different stroke? | Hoffa refers to repeating a stroke "three or four" times but sets up no definite routine | Suggestions for "three or four" strokes are included in descriptions. The number of strokes vary up to six and no set number is recommended | Mennell makes no reference to number of strokes to be given | The trend seems to be moving away from grouping strokes by numbers as indicated by the lack of mention of such in Mennell's text, and the fact that the majority of the people interviewed do not do so, except as a guide for beginners, which may have been all the basic texts meant it for |
| 16. Does return stroke always maintain contact? | Hoffa seems not to maintain contact with his return stroke | The hand should return to its original position without pressure but without losing contact with the part being massaged | The return stroke does not always maintain contact with the body, particularly with superficial stroking | McMillan's technique of maintaining contact on the return stroke is being used by most operators |
| 17. Do you ever "stroke off" a whole area, such as the back, the upper extremity, or the lower extremity? | No description of such a technique can be found in Hoffa's text | The back is stroked off when each division has been effleuraged and on the forearm as a final stroke | Mennell's "superficial stroking" is similar but of a superficial nature only | McMillan's influence has been felt in that the majority use this technique |

[a]The first column of Table 1 gives the questions asked; the second, third, and fourth columns explain, in brief, the methods of Hoffa, McMillan, and Mennell respectively; and the last column gives the conclusions derived from the questionnaire results.

TABLE 1-2. USE OF THE VARIOUS STROKES

| Question | Hoffa | McMillan | Mennell | Conclusions from Questionnaire Results |
|---|---|---|---|---|
| 1. Which of the effleurage strokes are used? | Hoffa describes the use of: light and deep stroking; knuckling; circular effleurage; thumb stroking; alternate-thumb stroking; simultaneous stroking | McMillan describes the use of: light and deep stroking; simultaneous stroking; alternate-hand stroking | Mennell describes the use of: superficial stroking; deep effleurage; simultaneous stroking | The majority of the operators use an effleurage that is predominantly the same, light and deep stroking, and simultaneous stroking. Alternate-hand stroking, which was mentioned by McMillan, is widely used as well as one-hand-over-the-other for deeper pressure. Also of note is the tendency for the operator to pick up Mennell's idea of superficial stroking, although they do not do it in the prescribed manner |
| 2. Which of the petrissage strokes are used? | Hoffa describes the use of petrissage which is: one-handed; two-handed (with flat hand for large flat surfaces and pick-up where possible); two-fingered | McMillan describes the use of petrissage which is: one-handed; two-handed; with alternate hands; finger and thumb; for small areas; flat-handed on the back | Mennell describes use of: kneading (circular movements in opposite directions); petrissage (raising muscle mass away from subjacent tissues); one-handed | Hoffa's techniques for petrissage are predominantly in use; McMillan's two-hand petrissage and Mennell's are very similar and this stroke is used by some |
| 3. Which of the friction strokes are used? | Hoffa describes the use of friction which uses: the thumb; the index finger; both thumb and index finger | McMillan describes the use of friction which uses: the thumb; two or three fingers; the thenar eminence | Mennell describes friction which uses any part of the hand, but especially the tips of the fingers or the balls of the thumbs | Use of the heel of the hand and one-over-the-other for pressure are not described by any of the basic texts, but are being used widely. Other techniques concerning friction are predominantly the same, except for the few people who com- |

| | Hoffa | McMillan | Mennell | Summary |
|---|---|---|---|---|
| | | | | bine friction and petrissage into a stroke that resembles both strokes |
| 4A. Is tapotement used routinely? B. Which of the tapotement strokes are used? | A. Tapotement is used routinely B. Hacking is the only tapotement stroke that is described | A. McMillan describes the use of tapotement routinely for a general massage B. Tapotement strokes described are: hacking; clapping; tapping; beating | A. Mennell describes the use of tapotement but does not use it routinely B. He describes the use of: hacking; clapping; beating | A. Whereas Hoffa used tapotement routinely and McMillan described its use in a general massage, Mennell states that he does not use it routinely and the majority of the people surveyed use it for certain pathologic conditions only. B. Use of the various strokes is fairly unified |
| 5. How is vibration used? | Hoffa does vibration either with the points of the fingers or with a flat hand but advises the use of a mechanical vibrator | McMillan describes vibration as being done with one finger or several and also with the flat hand | Mennell believes that the hand is a poor substitute for a mechanical vibrator | Although described by all three of the basic texts, it is used very little |
| 6. Which other strokes are used? | None | The five fundamental procedures can form the basis for a large variety of manipulations | Mennell describes "shaking" in which the hand grasps the part giving quick firm vibrations which shake it from side to side. He also mentions a stroke which is similar to friction, but it is applied in a transverse plane to the muscle fibers | Horizontal stroking for the low back is rather widely used although very few have a name for this stroke. Mennell's frictionlike stroke, which is done in a transverse plane, is used by some. Although used by only a few, Storms' technique for nodules has made some impression in this country |

# Suggestions for Practical Testing

Applications of massage techniques are difficult to evaluate, and grades are often subjective. Since people have the right to as accurate an evaluation as possible, the following chart (Fig. A–1) is suggested as a means to a numerical evaluation on which a grade can be given. Apparent weaknesses can also be noted.

With this form, the instructor can list an entire class on one page, making possible a comparison of all marks. There are 24 items to evaluate, each of which can be given a maximum score of four. This gives a numerical total of 96 and allows four points that can be subtracted or added under "remarks" for incidentals not listed among the other 24. These could be such things as "leaning on the patient," or "dragging a towel or sleeve across the part to be treated."

In this way, the instructor can justify the grade by showing a numerical mark. The form also provides a written record that can be reviewed with the teacher.

Some instructors may prefer a briefer form. Figure A–2 is a form that can be used for one person. This leaves more room for remarks than the one previously shown. It can also be evaluated numerically. To help the therapist know what the patient is thinking, he or she should ask leading questions such as the ones written in Figure A–3.

Name _____

Statement of Problem or Case:

| | GRADE | REMARKS |
|---|---|---|
| +10<br>Positioning | | |
| +10<br>Draping | | |
| +10<br>Choice and Use of<br>Lubricant | | |
| +20<br>Organization<br>Overall Approach | | |
| +20<br>Skill in<br>Technique | | |
| +10<br>Termination<br>Dressing, etc. | | |
| +20<br>Overall Impression | | |
| Final Grade | | |

**Figure A2-1.** Practical evaluation sheet for instructor's use in massage.

| Technique of Operator | Name of Operator | | | | | | | |
|---|---|---|---|---|---|---|---|---|
| Draping | | | | | | | | |
| Positioning | | | | | | | | |
| Effleurage, Rhythm | | | | | | | | |
| &#8243;     Pressure | | | | | | | | |
| &#8243;     Pattern | | | | | | | | |
| Petrissage, Rhythm | | | | | | | | |
| &#8243;     Pressure | | | | | | | | |
| &#8243;     Progression | | | | | | | | |
| Friction, Rhythm | | | | | | | | |
| &#8243;     Pressure | | | | | | | | |
| &#8243;     Pattern | | | | | | | | |
| Tapotement, Rhythm | | | | | | | | |
| &#8243;     Pressure | | | | | | | | |
| &#8243;     Pattern | | | | | | | | |
| Vibration | | | | | | | | |
| Other Strokes | | | | | | | | |
| Use of Lubricant | | | | | | | | |
| Posture | | | | | | | | |
| Condition of Hands | | | | | | | | |
| Personal Appearance | | | | | | | | |
| Knowledge of Case | | | | | | | | |
| Attitude, Poise | | | | | | | | |
| Overall Approach | | | | | | | | |
| Clean-Up | | | | | | | | |
| Remarks | | | | | | | | |
| Numerical Total | | | | | | | | |
| Final Grade | | | | | | | | |

GRADING KEY
A—Excellent      4
B—Above Average   3
C—Average        2
D—Below Average   1
F—Failing         0

Remarks

**Figure A2-2.** Practical evaluation sheet for instructor's use in massage.

In order to maximize the effectiveness and safety of massage sessions together, please take the time to carefully fill out this questionnaire. This information will be treated confidentially. Use back of page if extra space is needed. Your feedback is appreciated during and at the end of the sessions to help in tailoring the massage session to serve in the best possible way.

Name _____ Date of initial visit _____

Address _____ Referred by _____

Phone (day) _____ (eve) _____ Date of birth _____

Occupation(s) _____

Interest(s) _____

What is your goal/concern for today's session?

What is your previous experience with professional massage?

Do you experience any difficulty lying either on your front or your back?

Is there any area where you would like extra time spent, any area where you seem to hold a lot of tension?

Habits: Exercise _____
　　　　　Tobacco _____ Alcohol _____ Drugs (non-med.) _____
　　　　　Posture assumed most of day _____
　　　　　Sleep _____ Bowels _____ Caffeine _____

Medical History:
— Hypertension　　　— PMS/painful men-　　— Mental illness
— Heart disease　　　　struation　　　　　　— Osteoporosis
— Arteriosclerosis　　— Easy bruising　　　— Osteoarthritis
— Varicose veins　　　— Skin rash　　　　　— Rheumatoid arthritis
— Phlebitis　　　　　— Abscess or open　　— Fibrositis
— Epilepsy　　　　　　sore　　　　　　　　— Herniated disc
— Headaches　　　　— Skin sensitivity　　— Inner ear problem
— Cancer/malignancy　— Allergies　　　　　— Pregnancy
— Diabetes　　　　　— Herpes I or II

— Surgery/fractures (explain):

— Musculoskeletal pain/stiffness (such as low back, neck, shoulder, etc.) (explain)

— Any other physical or emotional difficulties? (explain)

Do you wear contacts ( ), dentures ( ), or hearing aid ( )?

Are you under medical care or supervision now? ( ) For what condition?

Are you currently taking any medication? ( ) If so, what?

Are there specific aspects of your life that are particularly stressful? (job, posture, habits, diet, family, etc)? (explain)

Do we have your permission to contact your physician should the need arise?

Name of Physician _____ Phone _____

Signature _____ Date _____

**Figure A2-3.** Client questionnaire.

# Bibliography

Academy of Traditional Chinese Medicine. (1975). *An outline of Chinese acupuncture.* Peking: Foreign Language Press. (Note: This is the most accurate text on acupuncture points that has been translated from the Chinese.)

Anhui Medical School Hospital/China. (1983). *Chinese massage therapy.* Boston: Shambhala Publications.

Armstrong, M. E. (1972, September). Acupuncture. *American Journal of Nursing,* 1582.

Auckett, A. D. (1981). *Baby massage.* New York: Newmarket.

Baloti, L. D. & Harrison, L. (1983). *Massageworks.* New York: Putnam.

Barstow, Cedar, M. (Ed.). (1985). *Tending body and spirit: Massage and counseling with elders.* Boulder, CO: Author.

Bauer, C. (1987). *Acupressure for women.* Freedom, CA: Crossing Press.

Beau, G. (1972). *Chinese medicine.* New York: Pyramid House.

Benjamin, B. E. (1978) *Are you tense? The Benjamin system of muscular therapy.* New York: Pantheon.

Benjamin, P. J. (1986, Summer). The seeds of a profession. *The Massage Journal, 41.*

Berkson, D. (1977). *The foot book: Healing the body through reflexology.* New York: Funk & Wagnalls.

Bohm, M. (1913). *Massage: Its principles and technic.* (Elizabeth Gould trans.) Philadelphia: Saunders.

Boone, J. A. (1954). *Kinship with all life.* New York: Harper & Row.

Byers, D. C. (1983). *Better health with foot reflexology.* Florida: Ingham Publishing.

Caldwell Brown, C. (Ed.). (1984). *The many facets of touch.* Skillman, NJ: Johnson & Johnson Baby Products Co.

Carnahan, B. (1985). *A gentle touch: Massage therapy for people in painful times.* Boulder, CO: Boulder County Hospice.

Cerney, J. V. (1974). *Acupressure, acupuncture without needles.* New York: Cornerstone Library.

Cousins, N. (1977, May 28). Anatomy of an illness (as perceived by the patient). *Saturday Review*, 4, 48.

Cousins, N. (1979). *Anatomy of an illness*. New York: Norton.

Cousins, N. (1983). *The healing heart*. New York: Norton.

Chaitow, L. (1980). *Neuro-muscular technique: A practitioner's guide to soft tissue manipulation*. London: Biddles.

Cyriax, J. & Russell, G. (1977). *Textbook of orthopaedic medicine*, Vol. II (9th ed.). London: Balliere Tindall.

deLangre, J. (1971). *The first book of do in, guide pratique Vol. 1*. Magalogia, CA: Happiness Press.

Dicke, E., Schliack, H., & Wolff, A. (1978). *A manual of reflexive therapy of the connective tissue "Bindegewebsmassage."* Germany: Sidney S. Simon.

Dicke, E. (1956). *Meine Bindegewebsmassage*. Stuttgart: Hippokrates-Verlag.

Downing, G. (1974). *The massage book*. New York: Random House; Berkeley, CA: Bookworks.

Ebner, M. (1962). *Connective tissue massage*. New York: Drieger.

Ebner, M. (1956, August). Peripheral circulatory disturbances: Treatment by massage of connective tissue reflex zones. *British Journal of Physical Medicine, 19*, 176.

Fulton, J. F. (1931). *A textbook of physiology*. Philadelphia: Saunders.

Gach, M. R. (1981). *The acupuncture stress management book, Acu-Yoga*. Tokyo: Japan Publications.

Goldstein, A. (1976, September 17). Opioid peptides (endorphins) in pituitary and brain. *Science, 193*, 1081.

Gordon, R. (1978). *Your healing hands; The polarity experience*. Santa Cruz, CA: Unity Press.

Grad, B. (1964). A telekinetic effect on plant growth, Part 2. Experiments involving treatment with saline stoppered bottles. *International Journal of Parapsychology, 6*, 473.

Graham, D. (1902). *Treatice on massage: Its history, mode of application and effects*. Philadelphia: Lippincott.

Greed, M. (1975). *The healing hand*. Cambridge, MA: Harvard University Press.

Green, E. & Green, A. (1973). The ins and outs of mind–body energy. *Science Year, 1974: World Book Science Annual*. Chicago: Field Enterprises.

Guarino, E. (1987, August 19). Manual lymphatic drainage. *The Physical Therapy Forum, VI*, 33.

Hashimoto, M. (1968). *Japanese acupuncture*, New York: Live right.

Head, H. (1920). *Studies in neurology*. London: Henry Frowde, Hodder & Stoughton.

Heinl, T. (1983). *The baby massage book*. New Jersey: Prentice-Hall.

Hoffa, A. J. (1978). *Technik der massage* (14th ed.). Stuttgart: Ferdinand Enke.

Huang, M. (1975). Medical seminar at Chinese acupuncture science research foundation. Taipei, Taiwan, R.O.C.

Ingham, E. D. (1959). *Stories the feet can tell: Stepping to better health*. Rochester, NY: Ingham Publishing.

Ingham, E. D. (1959). *Stories the feet have told*. New York: Ingham Publishing.

Inkeles, G. (1983). *Massage and peaceful pregnancy*. New York: Putnam.

Institute of Traditional Chinese Medicine of Hunan Province. (1974). *Barefoot doctor's manual* (translation of a Chinese instruction to certain Chinese health personnel). Washington, DC: US Dept. of Health, Education, and Welfare, DHEW Pub. No. (NIH) p. 75.

Jackson, R. (1977). *Holistic massage.* New York, London: Drake Publishers.

Jacobs, M. (1960, February). Massage for the relief of anatomical and physiological considerations. *Physical Therapy Review, 40,* 96.

John E. Fogarty International Center. (1975). Acupuncture anesthesia. (a translation of Chinese publication of the same title) DHEW Publ. No. (NIH) p. 75.

Joy, W. Brugh. (1976). *Joy's way.* Los Angeles: Tarcher, distributed by Houghton Mifflin, Boston.

Kao, F. F. & Kao, J. J. (1973). *Acupuncture therapeutics: An introductory text* (a compilation and trans. by F. F. Kao.) New Haven: Eastern Press.

Kaptchuk, T. J. (1983). *The web that has no weaver.* New York: Congdon & Weed.

Kaye, A. & Matchan, D. C. (1978). *Mirror of the body.* San Francisco: Strawberry Hill Press.

Kellog, J. H. (1929). *The art of massage.* Michigan: Modern Medicine.

Kerr, F. W. L. (1975, September 29). Conference at the University of Connecticut Health Center.

Kimber, D. C., Gray, C. E., Stackpole, C. E., & Leavell, L. C. (1961). *Textbook of anatomy and physiology* (14th ed.). New York: MacMillan.

Knaster, M. (1986, July). *The wholistic athlete.* Brooklyn, MA: East–West.

Kogan, D. (1980). *Your body works.* Berkeley, CA: And/Or Press and Transformations.

Krieger, D. (1976, April). Nursing research for a new age. *Nursing Times,* 1–7.

Kunz, K. & Kunz, B. (1984). *Hand and foot reflexology: A self-help guide.* New Jersey: Prentice-Hall.

Kunz, K. & Kunz, B. (1985). *Hand reflexology workbook.* New Jersey: Prentice-Hall.

Kurz, I. (1982). *Introduction to Dr. Vodder's manuel lymphatic drainage,* Vol I–II. (2nd ed.). Heidelberg: Haug Publishers.

Ladd, M. P. & Kottke, F. J. (1952). Studies of the effects of massage on the flow of lymph from the foreleg of the dog. *Archives of Physical Medicine, 3,* 604.

LaFreniere, J. G. (1984). *LaFreniere body techniques.* New York: Masson Publishing.

LeBoyer, F. (1976). *Birth without violence.* New York: Knopf.

Levine, S. (1982). *Who dies?* Garden City, NY: Anchor Press/Doubleday.

Lidell, L. (1984). *The book of massage.* New York: Simon & Schuster.

Manaka, Y. & Urquharth, I. A. (1972). *The layman's guide to acupuncture.* New York: John Westerhill.

Mann, F. (1973). *Acupuncture, the ancient Chinese art of healing and how it works scientifically.* New York: Vintage Books.

Mann, F. (1966). *Atlas of acupuncture, points and meridians in relation to surface anatomy.* London: William Heinemann Medical Books.

Mann, F. (1967). *The treatment of disease by acupuncture.* London: William Heinemann Medical Books.

Marquardt, H. (1983). *Reflex zone therapy of the feet.* (A. C. Lett, Trans.). New York: Thorson's Press.

Marx, J. L. (1976, September 24). Neurobiology: Researchers high on endogenous opiates. *Science, 193,* 1227.

Masunaga, S. & Ohashi, W. (1977). *Zen Shiatsu: How to harmonize Yin and Yang for better health.* New York: Japan Publications/Harper & Row.

McGarey, W. A. (1974). *Acupuncture and body energies.* Phoenix: Gabriel Press.

McMillan, M. (1932). *Massage and therapeutic exercise* (3rd ed.). Philadelphia: Saunders.

Meagher, J. (1986). *Beating muscle injuries for runners.* Springfield, MA: Jack Meagher.

Meagher, J & Boughton, P. (1980). *Sportsmassage*. Garden City, NJ: Dolphin Books.

Mennell, J. B. (1945). *Physical treatment by movement, manipulation and massage* (5th ed.). Philadelphia: Blakiston.

Montague, A. (1971). *Touching*. New York: Harper & Row.

Moor, F., Peterson, S., Manwell, E., et al. (1964). *Manual of hydrotherapy and massage*. CA: Pacific Press.

Mottice, M., Goldberg, D., Benner, E. K., & Spoerl, J. (1986). *Soft tissue mobilization techniques*. Ohio: JEMD Co.

Namikoshi, T. (1969). *Shiatsu: Health and vitality at your fingertips*. San Francisco: Japan Publications.

Namikoshi, T. (1974). *Shiatsu therapy theory and practice*. New York: Japan Publications.

Ohashi, W. (1976). *Do-it-yourself Shiatsu*. New York: Dutton.

Older, J. (1982). *Touching is healing*. New York: Stein & Day.

O'Regan, B. (1987, Spring). Inner mechanisms of the healing response. *Massage Therapy Journal, 50*, 21.

Osterbye, C. (1987). Baby massage. *Massage & Healing Arts Magazine, 2*, 28.

Palos, S. (1972). *The Chinese art of healing*. New York: Bantam.

Pfrimmer, T. C. (1970). *Muscles—Your invisible bonds*. New York: Vantage.

Phaigh, R. & Perry, P. (1984). *Athletic massage*. New York: Simon & Schuster.

Kurpian, W. (Ed.). (1981). *Physical therapy for sports*. Philadelphia: Saunders.

Porth, C. M. (1986). *Pathophysiology: Concepts of altered health states* (2nd ed.). Philadelphia: Lippincott.

Prudden, B. (1984). *Pain erasure*. New York: Evans.

Prudden, B. (1984). *Myotherapy: Bonnie Prudden's complete guide to pain-free living*. New York: Doubleday.

Rice, R. D. (1975, November). Premature infants respond to sensory stimulation. *American Psychological Association Monitor, 6*:11, 8.

Robbins, S. L., Cotran, R. S., & Kumar, V. (1984). *Pathologic basis for disease* (3rd ed.). Philadelphia: Saunders.

Rogers, P. (1977, April). Enkephalins. *Acupuncture Research Quarterly, 1*, 64.

Rogoff, J. B. (1980). *Manipulation, traction and massage* (2nd ed.). Baltimore: Williams & Wilkins.

Schneider, V. (1982). *Infant massage*. New York: Bantam.

Segal, M. (1976). *Reflexology*. N. Hollywood, CA: Wilshire.

Seidman, M. (1982). *Like a hollow flute: A guide to polarity therapy*. CA: Elan Press.

Serizawa, K. (1974). *Massage: The Oriental method*. San Francisco: Japan Publications.

Serizawa, K. (1976). *Tsubo, vital points for Oriental therapy*. Japan: Japan Publications.

Shultz, W. (1976). *Shiatsu, Japanese finger pressure therapy*. New York: Bell Publishing.

Siegel, A. (1986). *Life energy: The power that heals*. Bridport, Dorset, England: Prism Press/Colin Spooner.

Siegel, B. S. (1986). *Love, medicine & miracles*. New York: Harper & Row.

Snyder, S. (1977, November 28). The brain's own opiates. *Chemical and Engineering News*, 35.

Solomon, W. M. (1950, August). *What is happening to massage? Archives of Physical Medicine*, 121.

Stanford University Medical Center. (1977). The morphine within. *The Healing Arts, 7,* 7.

Starr, D. (1987, October). Surprising new uses for acupuncture. *American Health,* 62.

Steiger, B. (1982). *Kahuna Magic.* Rockport, MA: Para Research.

Stone, R. (1986). *Polarity therapy: The complete collected works.* Reno, NV: CRCS Publications.

Storms, H. D. (1944, September). Diagnostic and therapeutic massage. *Archives of Physical Medicine, 25,* 550.

Tan, L. T., Tan, M. Y-C., & Veith, I. (1973). *Acupuncture therapy: Current Chinese practice.* Philadelphia: Temple University Press.

Teeguarden, I. (1978). *Acupressure way of health: Jin Shin Do.* New York: Japan Publications/Harper & Row.

Teeguarden, I. M. (1987). *The joy of feeling: Bodymind® acupressure.* New York: Japan Publications/Harper & Row.

Thrash, A. & Thrash, C. (1981). *Home remedies, hydrotherapy, massage, charcoal and other simple treatments.* Alabama: Yuchi Pines Institute Health Education Dept.

Tompkins, P. & Bird, C. (1973). *The secret life of plants.* New York: Avon.

Travell, J. G. & Simons, D. G. (1983). *Myofascial pain and dysfunction: The trigger point manual.* Baltimore: Williams & Wilkins.

Trotter, R. J. (1987, January). The play's the thing. *Psychology Today, 21,* 27.

Tsay, R. C. (1974). *Textbook of Chinese acupuncture medicine, Vol. I; General introduction to acupuncture.* Wappingers Falls, NY: Association of New Chinese Medicine.

Veith, I. (1972). *The Yellow Emperor's classic of internal medicine.* University of California Press.

Wale, J. O. (1968). *Tidy's massage and remedial exercises.* Bristol, England: IOP Publishing.

Wallnofer, H. & Von Rottausher, A. (1972). *Chinese folk medicine.* New York: Signet.

Wang, J. (1977, July). Breaking out of the pain trap. *Psychology Today, 11:*78, 86.

Wei-P' Ing, W. (1962). *Chinese acupuncture.* (trans J. Lauier; P. M. Chancellor.) Rustington, Sussex, England: Health Sciences Press.

West, O. (1983). *The magic of massage.* New York: Putnam

Wittlinger, H., & Wittlinger, G. (1982). *Introduction to Dr. Vodder's manual lymphatic drainage, Vols. I & II.* Heidelberg: Karl F. Haug Verlag GmbH & Co.

Wood, E. & Becker, P. (1981). *Beard's massage* (3rd ed.). Philadelphia: Saunders.

Worsley, J. R. (1972). *Is acupuncture for you?* New York: Harper & Row.

Yamamoto, S. (1979). *Barefoot Shiatsu.* Japan: Japan Publications.

# Index